*Praise for*

# THE SUBTLE BODY COLORING BOOK

"*The Subtle Body Coloring Book* is intriguing and fun. It provides all of us with a brilliant and kinesthetic way to learn the energy systems of our bodies while also relaxing and enjoying ourselves."

**CHRISTIANE NORTHRUP, MD,** author of the *New York Times* bestsellers *Goddesses Never Age; Women's Bodies, Women's Wisdom;* and *The Wisdom of Menopause*

"When we live with an awareness of color, we live a more colorful life—we go from bland to vibrant, from lackluster to vital. Let yourself go full-spectrum through the conduit of creativity with this exciting *Subtle Body Coloring Book!*"

**DR. DEANNA MINICH,** author of *Whole Detox*

"Cyndi Dale once again brings highly esoteric and very subtle energy into the realm of play and learning. What better way to learn about these powerful systems than to engage the unconscious directly by means of art: colors, shapes, and play. Although the energy systems she describes transcend easy-to-categorize shapes and contours, Dale offers a way to begin to imagine these systems—and begin to feel and sense them within ourselves—by leading us into the creative, imaginal realm. From there, our inner artist can begin to sense what exists all around us, but is very difficult to pin down. This is a gift to students and teachers of subtle energy, and to anyone whose inner child is yearning for both advanced knowledge and a simple way to get there."

**LAUREN WALKER,** author of *Energy Medicine Yoga* and *The Energy Medicine Yoga Prescription*

"All those who need to understand the critical issue of energy anatomy can benefit from this great workbook."

**C. NORMAN SHEALY, MD, PhD,** founder and CEO, International Institute of Holistic Medicine

"Wow! Such a beautiful way to deeply learn about the subtle energy systems of humanity: meridians, chakras, and colors. Live, love, and learn with this experiential coloring book!"

**BRIGITTE MARS,** coauthor of *The Country Almanac of Home Remedies* and *The Home Reference to Holistic Health and Healing*

"*The Subtle Body Coloring* book is a wonderful, engaged way to learn more about the energy body and energy fields. I love that Cyndi Dale included so much information on auric fields as it is key to healing work, distance healing work, and everyday interaction in the world. I am a huge fan of this coloring book and will use it with my energy students."

**DR. ANN MARIE CHIASSON,** Arizona Center for Integrative Medicine at the University of Arizona and author of *Energy Healing*

"The 'field' of energy medicine has become a legitimate and serious focus of study within physics and health care. We are happy for this! And thanks to Cyndi Dale, we now have a new creative option for study and integration of the fascinating concepts of the human energy system beyond scientific articles and textbooks. A lovely complement between the art texts of Alex Grey's *Sacred Mirrors* and the intellectually oriented scientific literature, Cyndi and her artist colleague, Richard Wehrman, offer us both a FUN and meaningful method to further integrate our understanding of the mystery of our human being-ness! Through this fascinating and well-done coloring book, one finds a lovely balance between 'just enough' text to whet our left brain's appetite for information and an artistic plethora of black and white figures with their energy anatomy, which satisfies the right brain and awaits your colored pencils and individual creativity! I will happily share this with students, colleagues, friends, and kids of all ages!"

**CYNTHIA HUTCHISON, DNSC, RN, HTCP/I,** Educational Program Director, Healing Touch Program; owner of Boulder Healing Touch

"Cyndi Dale's *The Subtle Body Coloring Book* makes the learning of energy into a fun and adventurous journey! She uses different healing modalities from a variety of traditions, which provides us with a wonderful interactive overview and are cross-informational between each other. I strongly recommend this unique book!"

**ROBERT PENG,** author of *The Master Key*

"Exploring subtle realms of healing brings together multiple ways of knowing and being. This coloring book allows us to learn and engage our imaginations in ways that embrace our expanded consciousness— and in turn invites us to harness the furthest reaches of our healing capacities. Now, sharpen your colored pencils and have fun."

**MARILYN SCHLITZ, MA, PhD,** author of *Death Makes Life Possible*

"I am excited about sharing this book with my students and clients. It is a game-changer for those people looking to upgrade how they dance through this life, as it is a master playbook. True healing takes place in our subtle bodies where the deepest development of our souls can emerge. Coloring is a therapeutic, harmonic practice that naturally creates an unfolding of all aspects of our mind, body, and spirit. I love this tool!"

**DR. LIGHT MILLER,** Ayurvedic College for Well-Being

# THE
# SUBTLE BODY
## COLORING BOOK

## ALSO BY CYNDI DALE

**Books**

*Advanced Chakra Healing: Cancer: The Four Pathways Approach*

*Advanced Chakra Healing: Energy Mapping on the Four Pathways*

*Advanced Chakra Healing: Heart Disease: The Four Pathways Approach*

*Attracting Prosperity Through the Chakras*

*Attracting Your Perfect Body Through the Chakras*

*Beyond Soul Mates: Open Yourself to Higher Love Through the Energy of Attraction*

*Energetic Boundaries: How to Stay Protected and Connected in Work, Love, and Life*

*Kundalini: Divine Energy, Divine Life*

*Llewellyn's Complete Book of Chakras: Your Definitive Source of Energy Center Knowledge for Health, Happiness, and Spiritual Evolution*

*The Complete Book of Chakra Healing: Activate the Transformative Power of Your Energy Centers*

*The Everyday Clairvoyant: Extraordinary Answers to Finding Love, Destiny and Balance in Your Life*

*The Intuition Guidebook: How to Safely and Wisely Use Your Sixth Sense*

*The Journey After Life: What Happens When We Die*

*Llewellyn's Little Book of Chakras*

*The Littlest Christmas Star: A Parable About Love*

*The Spiritual Power of Empathy: Develop Your Intuitive Gifts for Compassionate Connection*

*The Subtle Body: An Encyclopedia of Your Energetic Anatomy*

*The Subtle Body Practice Manual*

*Togetherness: Creating and Deepening Sustainable Love* (with Andrew Wald and Debra Evans)

**Audio Programs**

*Advanced Chakra Wisdom: Insights & Practices for Transforming Your Life*

*Energy Clearing: Heal Energetic Wounds, Release Negative Influences, and Create Healthy Boundaries*

*Healing Across Time and Space: Guided Journeys for Your Past, Future, and Parallel Lives*

*Illuminating the Afterlife: Your Soul's Journey Through the World's Beyond*

**Video Programs**

*Cyndi Dale's Essential Energy Healing Techniques*

The *Songbird* series

*The Subtle Body Online Training Program*

# THE
# SUBTLE BODY
# Coloring Book

## Learn Energetic Anatomy—
## from the Chakras to the Meridians and More

.................

CYNDI DALE

Illustrated by
RICHARD WEHRMAN

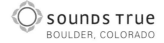

SOUNDS TRUE
BOULDER, COLORADO

Sounds True, Inc.
Boulder, CO 80306

This book is not intended as a substitute for the medical recommendations of
physicians, mental health professionals, or other healthcare providers. Rather, it is
intended to offer information to help the reader cooperate with physicians, mental
health professionals, and health providers in a mutual request for optimum well-
being. We advise readers to carefully review and understand the ideas presented and
to seek the advice of a qualified professional before attempting to use them.

Published 2017

Cover design by Rachael Murray
Book design by Lisa Kerans

Printed in South Korea

Library of Congress Cataloging-in-Publication Data
Names: Dale, Cyndi, author.
Title: The subtle body coloring book : learn energetic anatomy—from the chakras
    to the meridians and more / Cyndi Dale.
Description: Boulder, Colorado : Sounds True, 2017. |
    Includes bibliographical references.
Identifiers: LCCN 2016041165 | ISBN 9781622036073 (pbk.)
Subjects: LCSH: Energy medicine. | Chakras—Health aspects.
Classification: LCC RZ421 .D3513 2017 | DDC 615.8/52—dc23
LC record available at https://lccn.loc.gov/2016041165

10  9  8  7  6  5  4

*Actually, all education is self-education. A teacher is only a guide . . .*
*What you receive is like the outlines in a child's coloring book.*
*You must fill in the colors yourself.*

LOUIS L'AMOUR

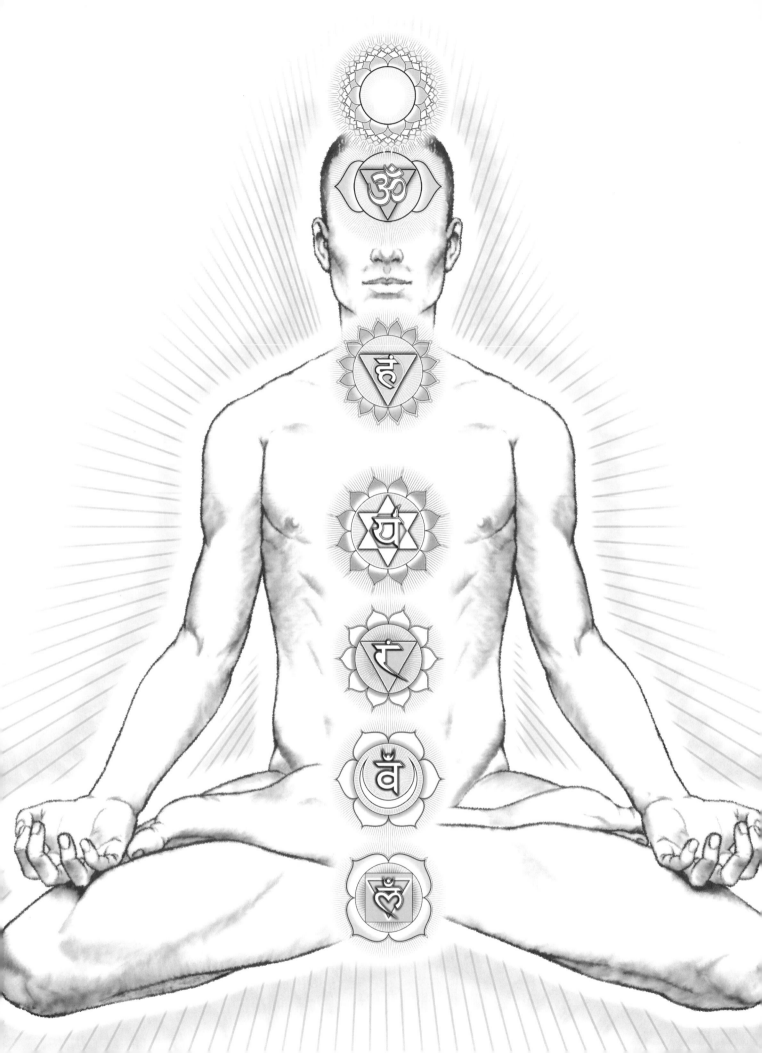

# CONTENTS

List of Illustrations . . . viii

Introducing *The Subtle Body Coloring Book* . . . 1

Part I   ENERGETIC FIELDS: VIBRATIONS OF LIGHT AND SOUND . . . 7

Part II   THE MERIDIAN SYSTEM: CHANNELS OF CHI . . . 23

Part III   CHAKRAS: ENERGY BODIES OF LIGHT . . . 65

Part IV   SUBTLE ENERGY POINTS . . . 97

Bibliography . . . 127

About the Author . . . 129

About the Illustrator . . . 130

# LIST OF ILLUSTRATIONS

*Introducing* **THE SUBTLE BODY COLORING BOOK**

0.1   First Chakra: Muladhara . . . 5

PART I   **ENERGETIC FIELDS: VIBRATIONS OF LIGHT AND SOUND**

1.1   Physical Fields of Light . . . 11

1.2   Subtle Energy Fields . . . 15

1.3   Layers of the Auric Field: The Seven-Layer Auric System . . . 19

1.4   Layers of the Auric Field: The Twelve-Chakra Auric System . . . 21

PART II   **THE MERIDIAN SYSTEM: CHANNELS OF CHI**

2.1   The Major Meridians: Front View . . . 31

2.2   The Major Meridians: Back View . . . 33

2.3   Lung Meridian: Tai Yin . . . 35

2.4   Large Intestine Meridian: Yang Ming . . . 37

2.5   Stomach Meridian: Yang Ming . . . 39

2.6   Spleen Meridian: Tai Yin . . . 41

2.7   Heart Meridian: Shao Yin . . . 43

2.8   Small Intestine Meridian: Tai Yang . . . 45

2.9   Bladder Meridian: Tai Yang . . . 47

2.10  Kidney Meridian: Shao Yin . . . 49

2.11  Pericardium Meridian: Jue Yin . . . 51

2.12  Triple Warmer Meridian: Shao Yang . . . 53

2.13  Gallbladder Meridian: Shao Yang . . . 55

2.14  Liver Meridian: Jue Yin . . . 57

2.15  Conception Vessel: Ren Mai . . . 59

2.16  Governor Vessel: Du Mai . . . 61

2.17  Head Meridians . . . 63

PART III   **CHAKRAS: ENERGY BODIES OF LIGHT**

3.1   Chakras and the Endocrine System . . . 73

3.2   The Hindu Chakra System . . . 75

3.3   First Chakra: Muladhara . . . 76

3.4   Second Chakra: Svadhisthana . . . 77

3.5   Third Chakra: Manipura . . . 78

3.6   Fourth Chakra: Anahata . . . 79

3.7   Fifth Chakra: Vishuddha . . . 80

3.8   Sixth Chakra: Ajna . . . 81

3.9   Seventh Chakra: Sahasrara . . . 82

3.10  The Three Main Nadis . . . 85

3.11  The Tibetan Six-Chakra System . . . 87

3.12  The Tsalagi (Cherokee) System . . . 89

3.13  Ojos de Luz: The Incan Energy System . . . 91

3.14  Incan Bands of Power Ritual . . . 93

3.15  The Twelve-Chakra System and Energy Egg . . . 95

PART IV   **SUBTLE ENERGY POINTS**

4.1   Basic Shiatsu Points: Side . . . 100

4.2   Basic Shiatsu Points: Back . . . 101

4.3   Basic Shiatsu Points: Front . . . 102

4.4   Keiketsu Shiatsu Points . . . 103

4.5   The Thai Energy System: Front . . . 105

4.6   The Thai Energy System: Back . . . 107

4.7   The Thai Energy System: Side . . . 109

4.8   Foot Reflexology: Top of the Foot . . . 111

4.9   Foot Reflexology: Sole of the Foot . . . 113

4.10  Foot Reflexology: Inner and Outer Left Foot . . . 115

4.11  Foot Reflexology: Inner and Outer Right Foot . . . 117

4.12  Hand Reflexology: Top of the Hand . . . 119

4.13  Hand Reflexology: Palm of the Hand . . . 121

4.14  Head Reflexology . . . 123

4.15  Auricular Reflexology . . . 125

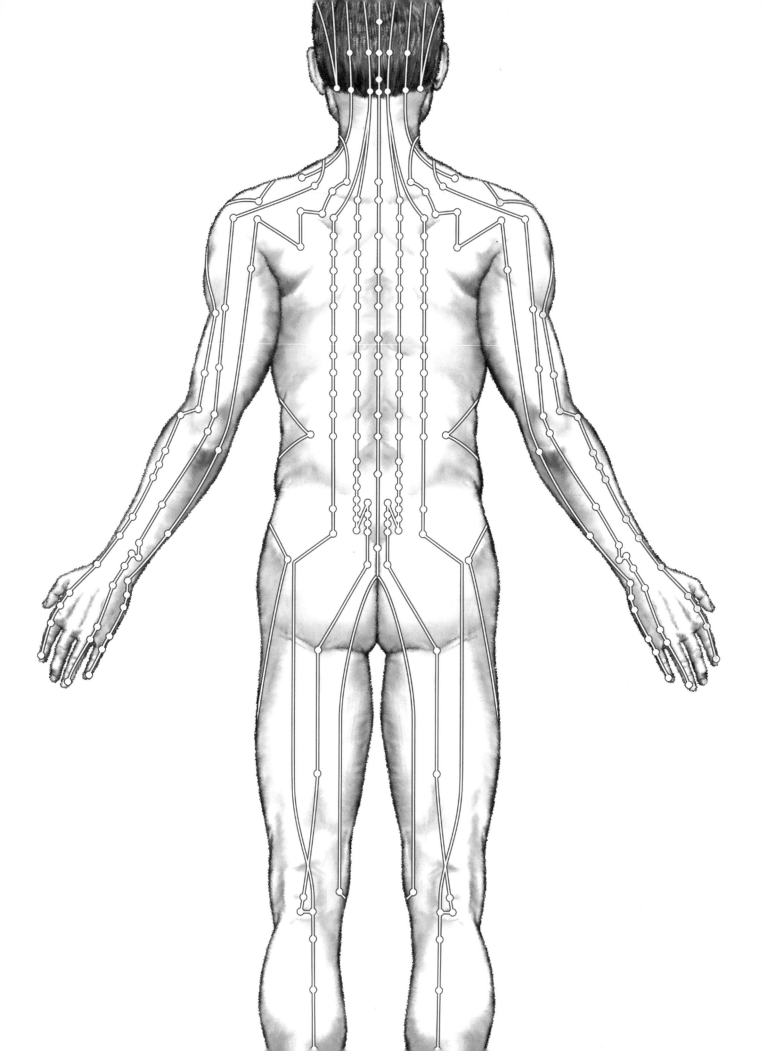

# *Introducing* THE SUBTLE BODY COLORING BOOK

Do you remember the delight you took in coloring when you were a child? How about the first time you used a camera and were able to explore your universe through snapshots? Remember how cool it was to cut out images from magazines for school reports or how fun—and messy—it was to craft new colors with finger paints?

Most teachings are presented verbally, but words can only go so far to explain the shapes, perceptions, feelings, and insights that make up reality. For a fuller understanding, we need images as well. The book this coloring book is based on, *The Subtle Body: An Encyclopedia of Your Energetic Anatomy*, employed both text and illustrations to teach on this wide-ranging topic. *The Subtle Body Practice Manual* added exercises for a direct experience of the energetic anatomy. Now, this coloring book aims to take your learning to a different level—the level of understanding you can gain by *interacting with images*. Or, put another way, by *playing* with images like you did when you were a kid.

More than anything, this book is a visual adventure, a colorful and gleeful journey to learning about the "you" within and beyond "you," as well as the other, complementary energies that construct this world. While much of your exploration will feel like play, the truth is that you will be learning with every stroke of the marker, pencil, or other instrument of your choice. And you will be educating yourself in one of the most effective and quickest of ways.

Most of us are kinesthetic learners. That means we learn by doing. What could be more active "doing" than coloring? Many of us are visual learners too. Hello, coloring fans! We also acquire new knowledge through verbalization and reading, so accompanying your expedition through the worlds of subtle energetics will be brief explanations that provide you with basic information about the images you are playing with. Just enough to get you oriented—the "main course" is coloring!

## THE SUBTLE ENERGY ANATOMY: A THUMBNAIL SKETCH

You already know that what you touch, see, taste, or hear is "real." Classical scientists prove their worth by defining and demonstrating the solidity of everything physical. Your favorite pie is made of measurable ingredients. Your liver has mass, and the air in your house is breathable. But in actuality, what composes everything concrete is invisible and inaudible. Even you—your body, thoughts, emotions, and soul—are a product of energy moving between the known and the unknown. In general, this coloring book will call the measurable energies "physical energy" and the immeasurable "subtle energy." The forms through which this energy flows inside and around you are collectively called the "subtle energy anatomy." It's the latter we are colorfully (and joyfully!) focusing on through this book.

## GET READY TO ILLUSTRATE THE SUBTLE WORLD!

### HOW THIS BOOK IS ORGANIZED

As you enter the colorful world of subtle energetic anatomy, you'll discover that there are three basic subtle energy structures: fields, channels, and centers. This book is orchestrated to help you explore these three structures as well as some of their offshoots. In Part I, you'll play with energetic fields, both physical and subtle. Then in Part II, you'll move into coloring the channels through which energy flows, learning about the meridians of Traditional Chinese Medicine. Part III gives you plenty of opportunity for hands-on learning about subtle energy bodies, with an emphasis on chakras—including a cross-cultural sampling of these—and *nadis*, the subtle channels related to the chakras. In Part IV, you will color subtle energy points, exploring various acupoints and other types of subtle points that empower healing and wellness. Finally, at the back of the book, you will find a list of references beyond *The Subtle Body: An Encyclopedia of Your Energetic Anatomy* and *The Subtle Body Practice Manual* to explore if you want to delve further into the world of subtle energy.

### YOUR COLORING SUPPLIES

Now it's time to get your coloring instruments figured out. For this endeavor, you'll want to select colored pencils that can be sharpened and/or fine-point colored markers. Why? Because some of the work is . . . subtle! It will be difficult to perform with crayons, chalk, or other thicker tools.

Your subtle artistry will be best served if you have these colors:

*The rainbow colors:* Medium to darker tones of red, orange, yellow, green, blue, indigo, and violet.

*Additional colors:* White, black, brown, pink, gray, silver, and gold. In addition to the blue and indigo in your rainbow set, you will want a light blue, too, so you can work with a range from dark to light. Also select a few additional pastel colors of your choice.

*Substitutions:* If you believe you'll have a hard time coloring with white, use lavender. If you can't obtain silver or gold colors, substitute a light gray and an orange-yellow, respectively.

## THE MEANINGS OF COLORS

In the world of subtle energy, colors hold specific energy. For some illustrations, certain colors are recommended because these colors carry meaning. For other illustrations, the colors you select are less important. This will be indicated as you move through the book.

If you choose to go "off road" and pick your own colors, the sidebar "What's in a Color?" will help you by giving you an overview of color theory. This more in-depth information will prove that coloring is, in and of itself, both an art and a science.

Following are a few insights about what the various colors or shades of color mean. These relate to the definition of energy as "information that moves or vibrates." In general, darker and deeper colors (colors with a deeper "value") are more physical and emotional in nature, and lighter colors are more spiritual and mental. This means that the effects colors have on your body, your psychology, and the world in general will be more physical or spiritual, respectively. Darker shades of a specific color will be apt to instigate immediate and powerful change, while lighter shades of that same color will evoke an uplifting or happy outcome. More specifically, these colors will usually generate the following responses in yourself or others:

*Red:* Passion and movement

*Orange:* Creativity and emotions

*Yellow:* Mentality and structure

*Green:* Healing and loving bonds

*Blue:* Overall, communication and knowledge. More specifically, *light blue* represents peace and infinity; *medium blue* conveys dependability and trustworthiness; *bright blue* stands for cleanliness and honesty; *deep blue* exemplifies strength of character; and *indigo*, a combination of blue and violet, epitomizes compassion and wisdom.

*Violet:* Strategic awareness and higher intuition

*White:* Purity and spirituality

*Gray:* Concealment and protection

*Black:* Mysticism and magic

*Brown:* Rootedness and naturalness

*Silver:* Openness to guidance; deflection of negativity

*Gold:* Integrity and spiritual power

Of course, there are many other colors, but these are the most basic, and they're all you will need in order

## WHAT'S IN A COLOR?

**LITTLE DID YOU** know that the simple act of coloring reveals the tip of a proverbial iceberg. The actual color we see, use, or select when coloring can be analyzed in a number of different ways. Knowing this information can help you select specific colors if you want to customize your colorations as well as gain insights into why the energetic systems explored in this book so frequently assign colors to certain structures. And why not impress yourself by being able to articulate what's going on in your artwork?

So you can best understand the following color concepts, it's recommended that you search "color wheel" on the Internet. You might even want to print a copy of a color wheel in full color and look at it when examining for the concepts explained next.

**The two ways to use color:** No matter how complicated or simple your coloring job, there are only two ways to put one or more hues together. These are contrast and harmony.

*Contrast* involves using colors that are dissimilar, meaning that there are no shared hues in the colors that make them up. We select contrasting colors when we want to generate a distinct impression, call attention to an image or message, or stimulate someone visually.

*Complementary colors* are an example of contrasting colors. These are direct opposites on a color wheel. Take a look at the color wheel that you found on the Internet and identify the opposites—red and green, yellow-green and red-violet, orange and blue, and so on. These are all complementary combinations with a strong impact.

*Harmony* employs colors that share similar hues and are found close together on the color wheel. Turn to your color wheel again and look for color harmonies. Red, red-orange, and orange all include red, for example, so are harmonious. When colors harmonize, they help the viewer feel soothed, calm, and pleased.

**Terms to color by:** There are specific terms that further define color. As you read through these, you might gain ideas about how to customize your color selections. For instance, at any time, you can tint an image, which involves adding white to your main color. Want to create a more somber impression? Use shading by adding black. Try it: you'll find that you can definitely feel the difference between a tint and a shade of a color.

*Primary colors:* All colors are made up from the three primary colors: red, blue, and yellow.

*Secondary colors:* Formed by mixing two primary colors.

*Tertiary colors:* Created by mixing a primary color with an adjacent secondary color. You can check out adjacent colors on the color wheel that you found on the Internet.

*Hue:* Another name for color.

*Tint:* A color plus white.

*Shade:* A color plus black.

*Tone:* A color plus gray.

As you can see, you've now greatly expanded your coloring vocabulary and selection choices. Go ahead and mix, match, tint, shade, tone, and more.

to playfully learn about the subtle body. Enjoy exploring how these colors make you feel as you are coloring in this book.

## HOW TO LEARN WHILE YOU COLOR

How can you best learn while you color? Know what color to use—and how? Here is some guidance:

- Background information is included for all of the illustrations in the book. It's bite-sized, so be sure to read it before you start coloring—start with the words, and then make the "music"!

- For text that is intended to be colored in, the letters will be hollow—or "bubbles."

- If that text is the title of a page, there may be specific recommendations for what colors to use. If there aren't, feel free to pick whatever color or colors you feel moved to use. If you want, select colors based on your mood, remembering that you can use shade, tint, and tone to further reflect your feelings.

- Color guidance: All illustrations include instructions for colors to use for each element on the page. You can use these colors to outline areas, fill them in, or both. Also feel free to use similar (harmonious) colors to outline and fill.

- Illustration labels or names: Some illustrations have simple labels that you will color, while others have those labels plus additional information to give you more context. Color all the words that have hollow letters, and refer to the associated information if you have questions about what you are coloring. The circles next to each label can be colored to make the visual association between the color, words, and location in the image.

- Structures: Dark lines depict the boundaries of various structures in the illustrations. You will color in the space between the boundaries, usually with the same color as the associated label.

## LET'S GET STARTED

Before sending you off on your coloring adventure, let's give you a chance to get your feet wet. On the facing page is a fairly simple illustration to get you started. This is *muladhara*, the first chakra in the Hindu system.

Now it's time to begin your coloring adventure in earnest. Enjoy learning as you create your own unique and beautiful subtle body imagery.

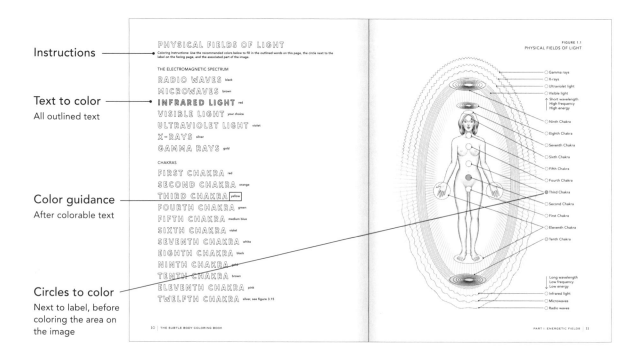

# FIRST CHAKRA: MULADHARA

Color: Red • Seed syllable: *Lam* • Element: Earth • Attribute: Patience • Granthi: Brahma

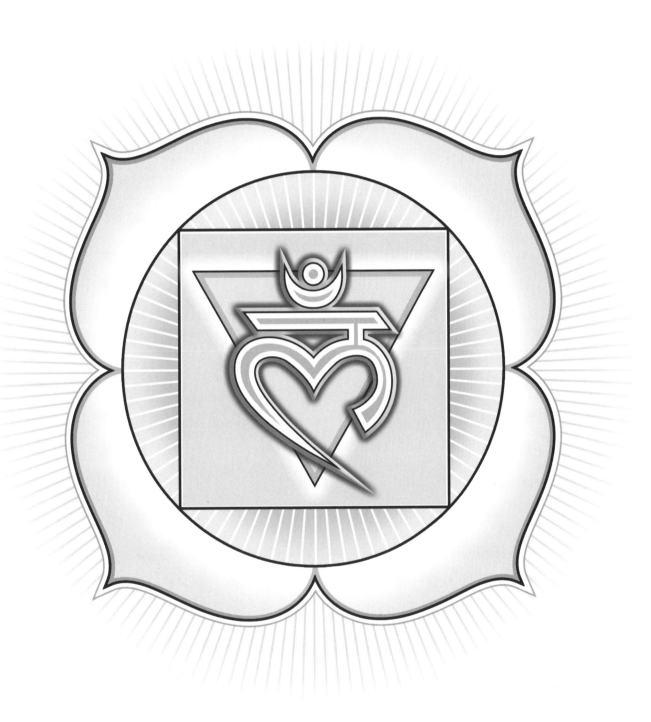

**FIGURE 0.1**

Coloring Instructions: Outline the square and triangle with gold. Also use gold to outline and fill in the mantra: the symbol within the square. Use red with a tint of yellow (to make vermilion) to color in the four lotus petals that surround the square. Fill in the remainder of the chakra and the label with red.

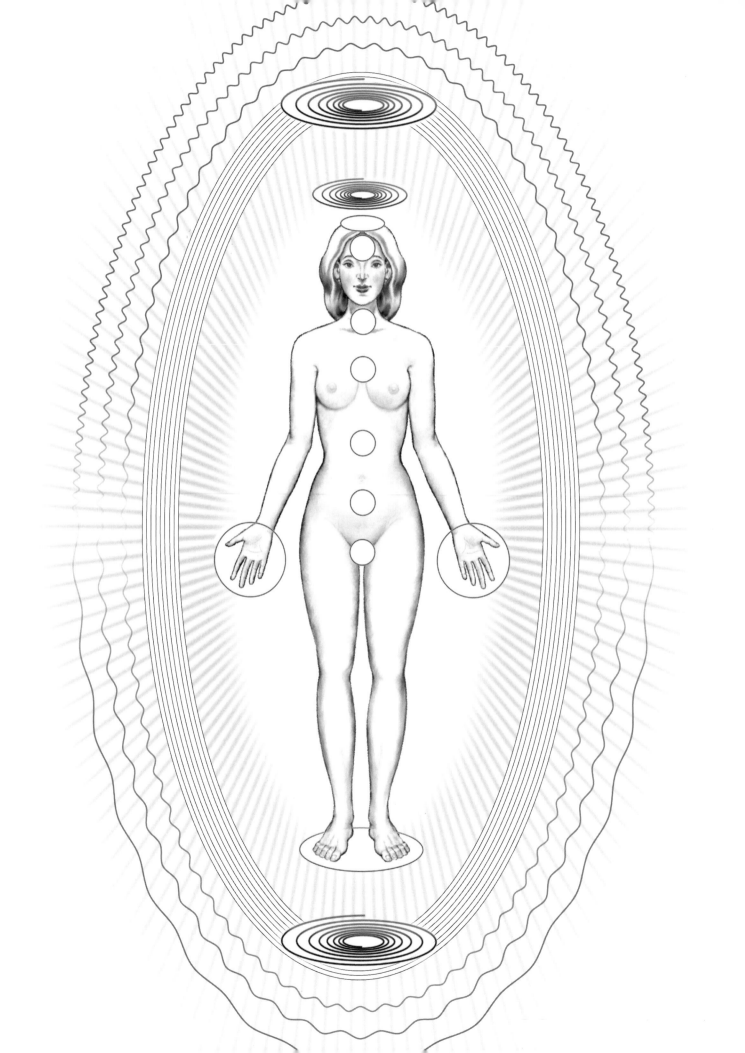

# PART I
## ENERGETIC FIELDS:
## VIBRATIONS OF LIGHT AND SOUND

Each of us (and the world) is made up of both measurable and subtle fields that create and sustain life. Measurable fields are also called *veritable fields*, and subtle fields are also named *putative fields*.

Classically, a field is an area in which a force exerts an influence at every point. Like all energetic structures, a field involves the vibration of energy and can carry information. Fields operate on both physical and subtle planes, as do energy bodies and channels. But fields present mysterious phenomena as well. Albert Einstein believed that the universe is composed of interconnected force fields, and recent physicists have pinpointed some of these fields as constructs of finite reality held within a greater infinity. Because of fields, reality is both local (or here and now) and nonlocal—occurring elsewhere and at other times. This means that everything across time and space is interconnected.

All fields interact, creating both beneficial and harmful effects on living organisms. Fields that are obvious to the senses interact with those that are hidden from the senses. The primary difference between physical and subtle fields is often simply the speed of the information and vibration involved. At some level, physical and subtle fields can actually be perceived as the same fields—one flowing into another, one creating and sustaining the other.

Fields exist everywhere. Each of us produces countless energy fields and interacts with endless numbers of external fields. Both measurable and subtle fields emanate from every cell, organ, and organ system, as well as from the entirety of our bodies. The same statement can be made in relation to all other living beings on this planet. In fact, the Earth itself and other planetary objects emit fields. Humans also create fields by manufacturing technological products; power lines and cell phones are two common examples. Even our subtle energy structures, like the chakras, radiate fields.

In order to best understand the complexity of fields, it's helpful to understand that there are three basic types, all of which are featured in this section:

1. Physical fields—also called veritable or measurable

2. Subtle fields—also called putative, representing fields that we're still learning how to measure

3. Auric fields—subtle energy layers that emanate from and surround the body

## PHYSICAL FIELDS: THE VERITABLE FIELDS WE CAN MEASURE

We are made of innumerable fields, all of which interact to shape, direct, and form our lives. The veritable or measurable energy fields are physical in nature and include sound and electromagnetic forces, such as visible light, magnetism, monochromatic radiation, and rays from the electromagnetic spectrum. Our body produces or is affected by all of these energies.

The chief field that generates and perpetuates life is the *electromagnetic spectrum*. The other life-sustaining category is *sound fields*, also called sound or sonic waves. Each part of the electromagnetic spectrum manifests as radiation that vibrates at a specific rate and therefore is called *electromagnetic radiation*. Our bodies require a specific amount of each part of this spectrum for optimal physical, emotional, and mental health. We can become ill or imbalanced if exposed to too much or too little of any particular stratum from the spectrum.

Yes—you are made of light! Electromagnetic radiation is described as a stream of photons, the wave-particles that are the basis of light. There are seven main types of electromagnetic radiation, each of which varies in wavelength, frequency, and energy. *Low energy* and *high energy* simply describe the information or energy of the photons, measured in electron volts. *Wavelength* is a way to measure the distance between two points on a wave. *Frequency* is the number of times waves cycle per unit of time.

The basic premise of physical electromagnetism is this: electricity generates magnetism. The most classical understandings depend on the fact that when electricity or charged electrons flow in a current, they create a magnetic field. These forces of electricity and magnetism together form electromagnetism. The reverse is also true: a changing magnetic field can create an electrical field.

Sound waves are the other major type of measurable wave. They are considered mechanical waves. Sound waves both affect us as human beings and emanate from us. While we don't feature them in this section, it's important to know that sound waves run at specific vibrations and penetrate all of existence. We can hear some sounds and not others, but that does not mean that the inaudible sounds do not affect us. These and other mechanical waves affect us either positively or negatively.

Fields of measurable electromagnetic radiation operate at levels we seldom perceive, yet they affect us nonetheless. Thus, the illustration (on page 11) of the physical fields combines veritable fields with chakras, which fall in the putative category. It depicts the twelve-chakra system (also featured on page 95), which includes in-body chakras as well as those extending beyond the physical body. The illustration reflects the fact that chakras, auric fields, and other subtle anatomy structures frequently interact with the measurable fields that we cannot see or hear.

*See pages 10–11 for Physical Fields of Light.*

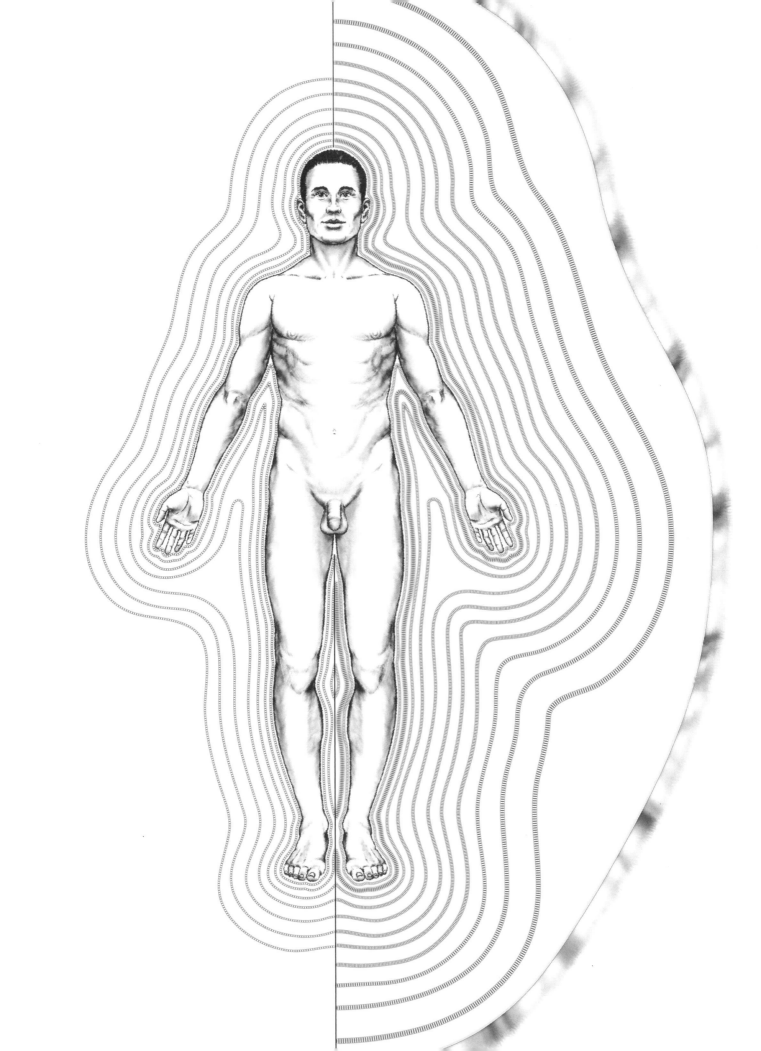

# PHYSICAL FIELDS OF LIGHT

Coloring Instructions: Use the recommended colors below to fill in the outlined words on this page, the circle next to the label on the facing page, and the associated part of the image.

## THE ELECTROMAGNETIC SPECTRUM

RADIO WAVES black

MICROWAVES brown

INFRARED LIGHT red

VISIBLE LIGHT your choice

ULTRAVIOLET LIGHT violet

X-RAYS silver

GAMMA RAYS gold

## CHAKRAS

FIRST CHAKRA red

SECOND CHAKRA orange

THIRD CHAKRA yellow

FOURTH CHAKRA green

FIFTH CHAKRA medium blue

SIXTH CHAKRA violet

SEVENTH CHAKRA white

EIGHTH CHAKRA black

NINTH CHAKRA gold

TENTH CHAKRA brown

ELEVENTH CHAKRA pink

TWELFTH CHAKRA silver, see figure 3.15

**FIGURE 1.1**
PHYSICAL FIELDS OF LIGHT

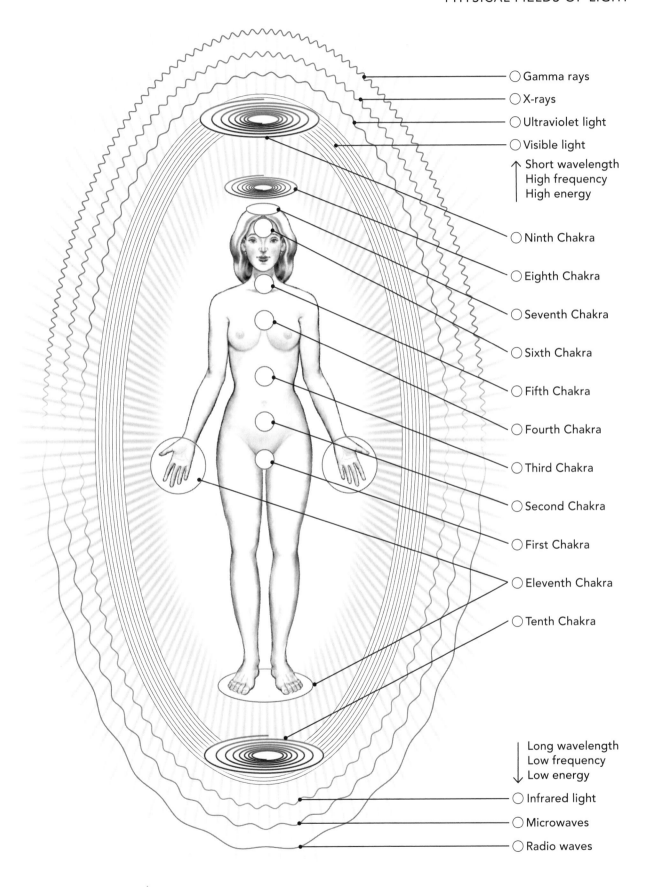

Gamma rays

X-rays

Ultraviolet light

Visible light

↑ Short wavelength
High frequency
High energy

Ninth Chakra

Eighth Chakra

Seventh Chakra

Sixth Chakra

Fifth Chakra

Fourth Chakra

Third Chakra

Second Chakra

First Chakra

Eleventh Chakra

Tenth Chakra

Long wavelength
Low frequency
↓ Low energy

Infrared light

Microwaves

Radio waves

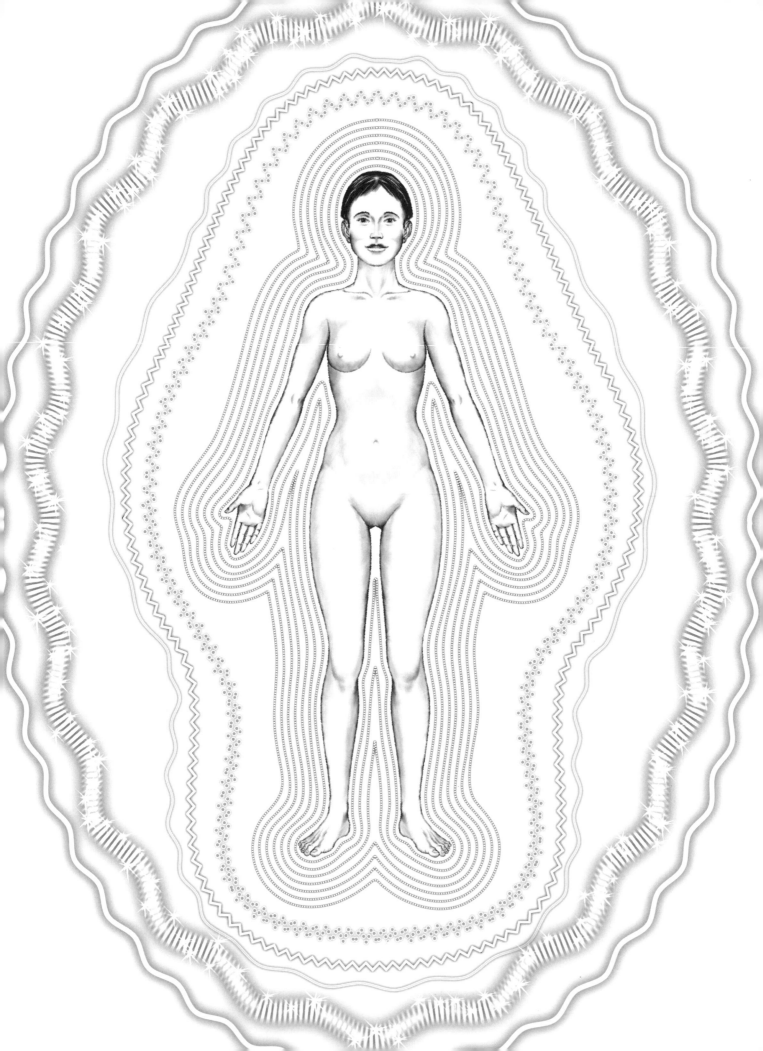

## SUBTLE ENERGY FIELDS

Subtle energy fields are also called *putative fields* or *biofields.* They are considered immeasurable, although modern science is starting to prove the existence of many of them. These fields explain the presence of vital life energy, called *chi* or *prana* in Asian cultures, as well as the sometimes extraordinary phenomena often labeled psychic, intuitive, or spiritual.

These energy fields are not separate from the mechanical or measurable fields; rather, they occupy a space and run at frequencies that cannot easily be perceived except through their effects. They are connected into the body by subtle energy channels such as the meridians and nadis, and subtle energy bodies, including the chakras, which are able to convert the fast-moving frequencies (chi and prana) into the slower and mechanical fields and forces (electricity, magnetism, and sound, among others). The energy channels and bodies are therefore "antennae" that receive and send information via the fields and transform this information for use by the body.

There are untold numbers of subtle fields. Several are depicted on page 15, for your coloring pleasure, and are described here.

**Auric field:** Part of the human energy field composed of a set of energy bands that graduate in frequency and color as they move outward from the body. Each auric field opens to different energy planes and energy bodies and also partners with a chakra, thus exchanging information between the worlds outside and inside of the body.

**Morphological field:** Fields that allow exchange between like-minded species and transfer information from one generation to another.

**T-field:** Subtle magnetic fields (also called thought fields) that allow the sharing of thoughts or psychic impressions. Comparable to consciousness. These steer L-fields.

**L-field:** Subtle electrical fields (also called life fields) that serve as a blueprint for life. They operate as a template for a developing organism.

**Universal field:** Also called a zero-point field, consisting of photons or units of light that regulate every living thing. Our DNA is made of light, and we are surrounded in a field of light; thus, the microcosm and macrocosm dance together.

**Geofields:** Earth- and cosmological-based fields that act upon all living organisms.

*See pages 14–15 for Subtle Energy Fields.*

# SUBTLE ENERGY FIELDS

Coloring Instructions: Use the recommended colors below to fill in the outlined words on this page, the circle next to the label on the facing page, and the associated part of the image.

## AURIC FIELDS

FIRST AURIC FIELD red

SECOND AURIC FIELD orange

THIRD AURIC FIELD yellow

FOURTH AURIC FIELD green

FIFTH AURIC FIELD medium blue

SIXTH AURIC FIELD violet

SEVENTH AURIC FIELD white

## ADDITIONAL FIELDS

MORPHOLOGICAL FIELD black

T-FIELD silver

L-FIELD pink

UNIVERSAL FIELD gold

GEOFIELDS brown

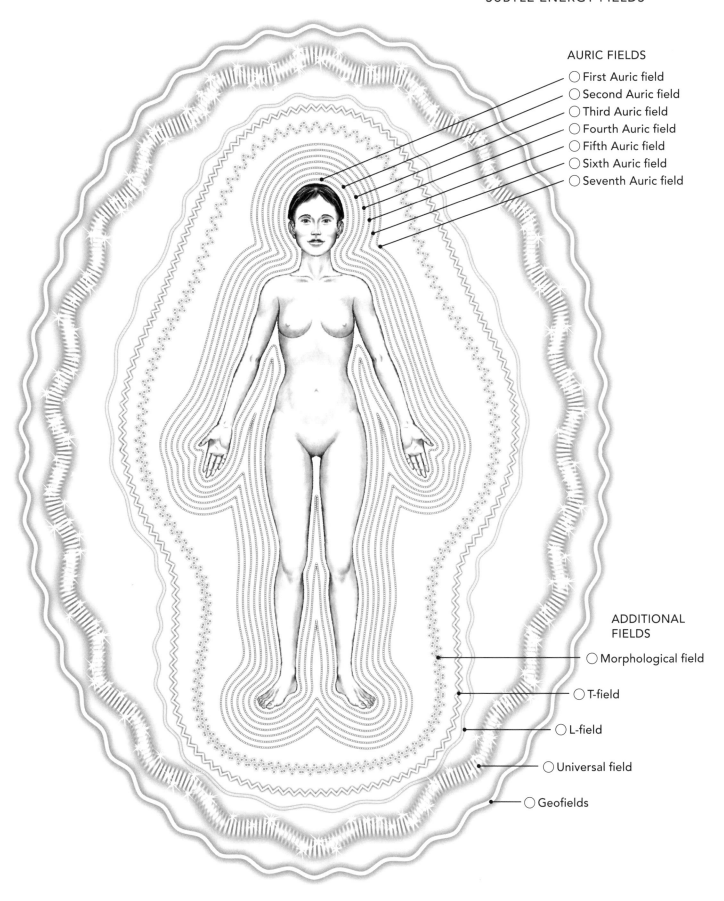

FIGURE 1.2
SUBTLE ENERGY FIELDS

AURIC FIELDS

○ First Auric field
○ Second Auric field
○ Third Auric field
○ Fourth Auric field
○ Fifth Auric field
○ Sixth Auric field
○ Seventh Auric field

ADDITIONAL
FIELDS

○ Morphological field

○ T-field

○ L-field

○ Universal field

○ Geofields

## LAYERS OF THE AURIC FIELD

Scientists have been investigating—and substantiating—the existence of the aura, the field that surrounds the entire body, for more than a hundred years, adding to the knowledge our ancestors already possessed. This field consists of multiple bands of energy, called *auric layers* or *auric fields*, that encompass the body, connecting us to the outside world.

There are many theories about the auric field, but most reveal the aura to have a fluid or flowing state; to be made up of different colors and therefore frequencies; to be permeable and penetrable; and to be magnetic in nature, although it also has electromagnetic properties. It is also reflective of the inner sanctum of the human being: the condition of it in general as well as its specific layers, reflecting the connections between subtle and physical energies as well as emotional and mental energies.

A special form of photography is actually able to take pictures of the auric field. In the 1930s, Russian scientist Semyon Kirlian and his wife, Valentina, invented a new photographic process that involves directing a high-frequency electrical field at an object.

The object's pattern of luminescence—the auric field—can then be captured on film. Contemporary practitioners are using Kirlian photography, among other special methods, to show how the aura responds to different emotional and mental states, and even to diagnose illness and other problems.

Besides the auric field, there are many other bands of energy that interpenetrate or surround the body. These might be called *energy bodies* or *energy planes*, and their names vary according to culture and system. In general, however, these fields are "stairsteps" that link the physical body to higher states. Barbara Ann Brennan, for instance, compartmentalizes seven auric layers into three planes, each of which represents an aspect of the human being. Each of these auric layers also has seven chakras within it. (For more information, please see Barbara Ann Brennan's book *Hands of Light*.)

The following pages showcase two depictions of the auric field. On pages 18–19 is Barbara Ann Brennan's assessment of the seven major auric layers, and pages 20–21 feature the aura of the twelve-chakra system.

**ON THE FOLLOWING** pages, fill in the outlined text and fields with the recommended colors below.

## THE SEVEN-LAYER AURIC SYSTEM

| COMPONENT OF AURA | DEFINITION | COLOR |
|---|---|---|
| **Spiritual plane** | **Manages spiritual realms** | Silver |
| Ketheric body | Reflects higher ideas | Gold |
| Celestial body | Holds higher emotions | Pastel of your choice |
| Etheric template | Blueprint for the etheric body / physical body | Deep Blue / Indigo |
| **Astral plane** | **Transforms physical and spiritual energies** | Silver |
| Astral body | Creates bonds | Pink |
| **Physical plane** | **Processes the physical world** | Brown |
| Mental body | Organizes thoughts | Yellow |
| Emotional body | Reflects emotions | Orange |
| Etheric body | Shapes the physical body | Light Blue |

## THE TWELVE-CHAKRA AURIC SYSTEM

| COMPONENT OF AURA | DEFINITION | COLOR |
|---|---|---|
| First auric field | Protection of life energies, passion | Red |
| Second auric field | Screens feelings and reflects emotions | Orange |
| Third auric field | Filters ideas and beliefs | Yellow |
| Fourth auric field | Attracts and repels relationships | Green |
| Fifth auric field | Attracts, repels, and sends guidance | Medium Blue |
| Sixth auric field | Opens to choices; enacts decisions | Violet |
| Seventh auric field | Connects with spirits and Spirit; broadcasts spiritual decisions | White |
| Eighth auric field | Broadcasts karma and absorbs power | Black |
| Ninth auric field | Connects with others based on soul issues | Gold |
| Tenth auric field | Mirrors beliefs; template for physical body | Brown |
| Eleventh auric field | Commandeers forces | Pink |
| Twelfth auric field | Connects to heavens; blends human and divine selves | Gray |

# THE SEVEN-LAYER AURIC SYSTEM

Coloring Instructions: Use the recommended colors below to fill in the outlined words on this page, the circle next to the label on the facing page, and the associated part of the image.

## SPIRITUAL PLANE silver
### MANAGES SPIRITUAL REALMS

## KETHERIC BODY gold
### REFLECTS HIGHER IDEAS

## CELESTIAL BODY pastel color, your choice
### HOLDS HIGHER EMOTIONS

## ETHERIC TEMPLATE deep blue/indigo
### BLUEPRINT FOR THE ETHERIC & PHYSICAL BODY

## ASTRAL PLANE silver
### TRANSFORMS PHYSICAL & SPIRITUAL ENERGIES

## ASTRAL BODY pink
### CREATES BONDS

## PHYSICAL PLANE brown
### PROCESSES THE PHYSICAL WORLD

## MENTAL BODY yellow
### ORGANIZES THOUGHTS

## EMOTIONAL BODY orange
### REFLECTS EMOTIONS

## ETHERIC BODY light blue
### SHAPES THE PHYSICAL BODY

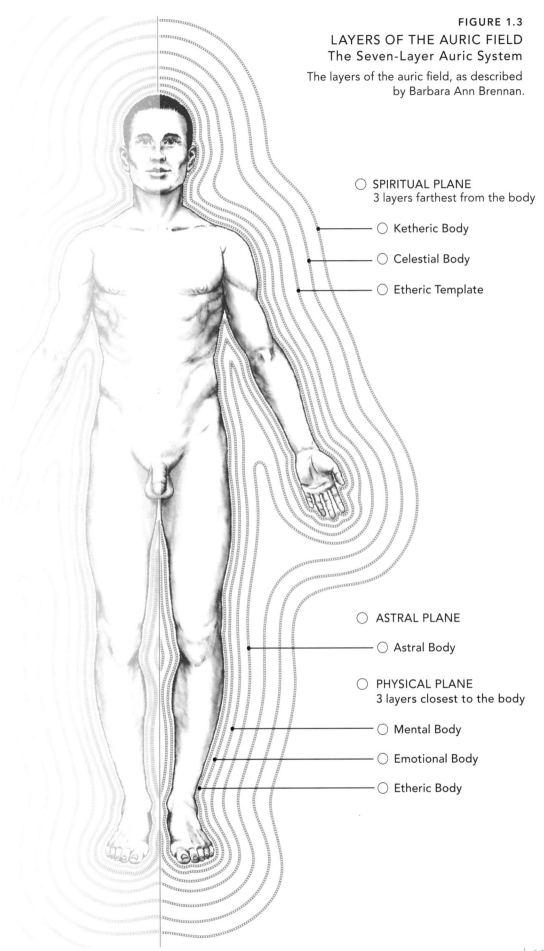

FIGURE 1.3
## LAYERS OF THE AURIC FIELD
### The Seven-Layer Auric System
The layers of the auric field, as described by Barbara Ann Brennan.

○ SPIRITUAL PLANE
3 layers farthest from the body

— ○ Ketheric Body

— ○ Celestial Body

— ○ Etheric Template

○ ASTRAL PLANE

— ○ Astral Body

○ PHYSICAL PLANE
3 layers closest to the body

— ○ Mental Body

— ○ Emotional Body

— ○ Etheric Body

# THE TWELVE-CHAKRA AURIC SYSTEM

Coloring Instructions: Use the recommended colors below to fill in the outlined words on this page, the circle next to the label on the facing page, and the associated part of the image.

## FIRST AURIC FIELD red
PROVIDES PRIMAL PROTECTION

## SECOND AURIC FIELD orange
FILTERS EMOTIONS

## THIRD AURIC FIELD yellow
SCREENS IDEAS

## FOURTH AURIC FIELD green
MANAGES RELATIONSHIPS

## FIFTH AURIC FIELD medium blue
GOVERNS GUIDANCE

## SIXTH AURIC FIELD violet
ACCESSES CHOICES

## SEVENTH AURIC FIELD white
CONNECTS SPIRITUALLY

## EIGHTH AURIC FIELD black
EMPOWERS KARMA

## NINTH AURIC FIELD gold
HARMONIZES SOULS

## TENTH AURIC FIELD brown
REVEALS ALL ISSUES

## ELEVENTH AURIC FIELD pink
COMMANDEERS FORCES

## TWELFTH AURIC FIELD gray
MAKES HEAVENLY BONDS

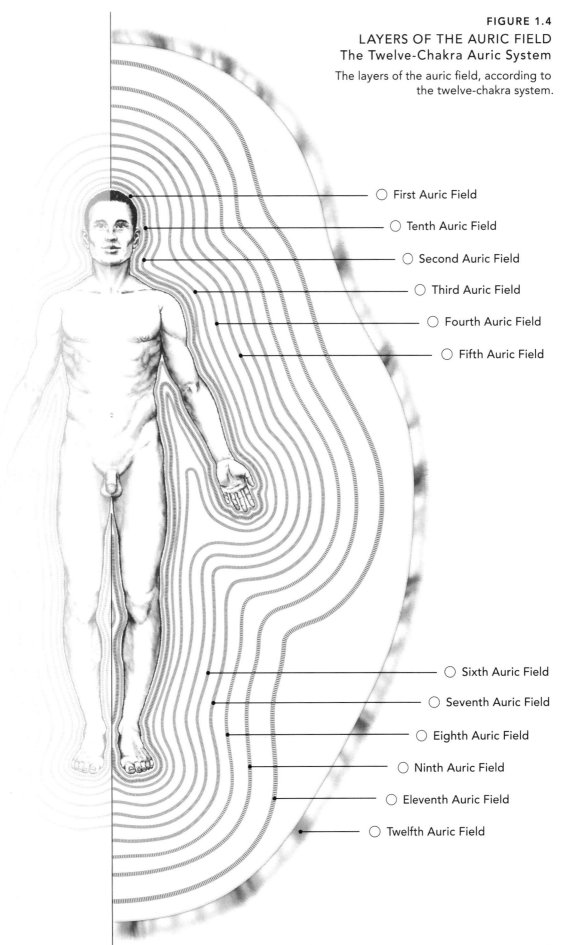

**FIGURE 1.4**
LAYERS OF THE AURIC FIELD
The Twelve-Chakra Auric System
The layers of the auric field, according to
the twelve-chakra system.

○ First Auric Field

○ Tenth Auric Field

○ Second Auric Field

○ Third Auric Field

○ Fourth Auric Field

○ Fifth Auric Field

○ Sixth Auric Field

○ Seventh Auric Field

○ Eighth Auric Field

○ Ninth Auric Field

○ Eleventh Auric Field

○ Twelfth Auric Field

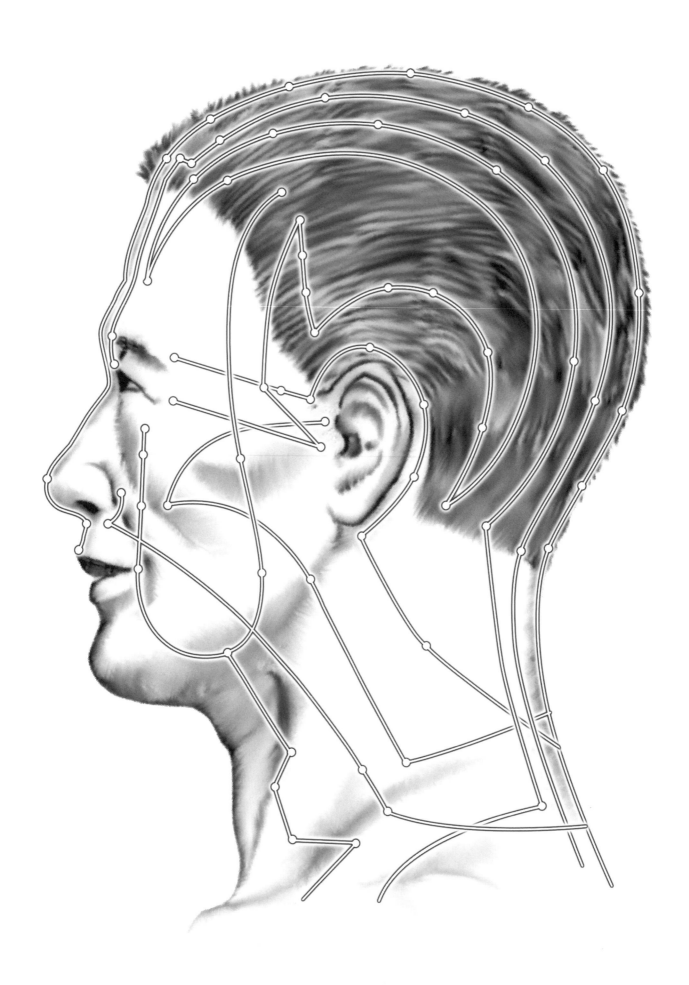

## PART II

# THE MERIDIAN SYSTEM: CHANNELS OF CHI

More than five thousand years ago, the Chinese discovered *meridians*, a set of subtle channels flowing through the body that are like rivers of energy—or rivers of light. This knowledge led to Traditional Chinese Medicine (TCM), the basis of many forms of Eastern medicine. The treatment modalities that utilize these channels include acupuncture, acupressure, and qi gong. All of these assist in the circulation of chi, the subtle energy that animates and informs everything, the energy required for life.

Traditional meridian therapy draws on these rivers of energy as well as the *five-phase theory*, which expresses that everything reduces to five basic elements: earth, metal, water, wood, and fire. Other concepts include *yin* (feminine earth energy) and *yang* (masculine heaven energy); the flow of emotions—joy, anger, grief, overthinking, and fear; the internal and external sources of disease; and the cyclical order of life as revealed in the cycles of the seasons.

These concepts have been carried into the descriptions of the meridians in this section of the coloring book. Every major meridian is either yin or yang in nature; relates to an emotion, an element, and a season; and is dominant for two hours out of every twenty-four-hour cycle. It is also partnered with a polar opposite, a meridian that is twelve hours apart in the twenty-four hour cycle. You'll learn these aspects of the meridians while you are coloring.

*Note: This introductory information will help you understand the illustrations throughout Part II.*

## THE MAJOR MERIDIANS

There are twelve major meridians, but these aren't the only meridians in the body. You'll meet members of two additional groups, including a few divergent meridians that emerge from the main meridians, as well as two of the *eight extraordinary channels*, which connect the main meridians. Specifically, you will locate and color the Governor vessel and the Conception vessel.

The twelve standard meridians run on the surface of the body, either on the chest, back, arms, or legs. They are the Lung, Large Intestine, Stomach, Spleen, Heart (sometimes called the Pericardium or Heart Protector), Small Intestine, Urinary Bladder, Kidney, Pericardium, Triple Warmer (sometimes called the Triple Burner, Triple Heater, or Three Heater), Gallbladder, and Liver. These terms refer to biological functions and not structural organs; however, all but the Triple Warmer and Heart meridians are connected to a specific organ system.

Altogether, the meridians are associated with more than four hundred acupuncture points (some sources count one thousand points), which are like "doorways" into the meridians. These are usually depicted with the abbreviation of the meridian, a number that signifies the point, and a particular name that is descriptive of its functions. Many acupoints are also linked with an element.

## IMPORTANT ACUPOINTS

The following acupoints are featured here in Part II. Also listed are the colors you'll be using to color in the points in this book. You will be coloring in the types of acupoints, using the colors indicated.

**Alarm points (Red):** Also called Mu points. Stimulating these points affects the organ but also its associated meridian. Often used to treat pain or excess energy.

**Associated points (Blue):** Also called Back Shu points. Positioned along the back of the body, these generally provide calm and are often used for chronic conditions.

**Shu points (Green):** Five important points that transport chi and relate to one of the five phases/ elements.

**Jing-well points (Gray):** Where the chi bubbles up. Helpful to restore consciousness, clear blocked energy all the way to the polar meridian, smooth mental anxiety, release heat, and benefit the spirit.

**Ying-spring points (Orange):** Where the chi glides down the channel. Working this point clears heat from the meridian and organ; known for clearing the complexion.

**Shu-stream points (Brown):** Where the chi pours through the channel; good for heaviness in the body and pain in the joints.

**Jing-river points (Yellow):** Where the chi flows down the channel. Helpful for lung issues, for example.

**He-sea points (Black):** Where the chi collects to travel deeper into the body. Benefits stomach and skin issues.

**Yuan-source points (Light Blue):** Releases chi and benefits internal organs, often releasing issues at their causal level.

**Cardinal points (Silver):** Also called Empirical points, 360 points specific to conditions, functions, and areas of the body.

**Xi-cleft points (Pink):** Stimulates flow of chi if it has accumulated, alleviating chronic conditions and pain.

**Luo-connecting points (Violet):** Where the main meridians converge and communicate with each other.

Healers work with the meridians and acupoints in many ways. Treatments include *acupuncture*, the use of needles to stimulate the meridians through the acupoints; *acupressure*, the stimulation of points through massage, fingers, or even elbows; *cupping*, which involves applying glass cups to the skin near the meridians, using suction to stimulate the flow of energy; and *electrodermal screening* and other uses of computerized and electrical equipment to diagnose and stimulate the points. Points are also stimulated with tools including color, magnets, sound, stones, tuning forks, and more.

## YOUR MERIDIAN ABBREVIATIONS AND COLORS

The main meridians are numbered 1 through 12, with two secondary meridians numbered 13 and 14. There are several different abbreviation shorthands. I've described one commonly used system, which is used for this coloring book. And because this book is all about *coloring*, I've also provided a list of the colors assigned to the meridians. The colors will also be repeated on the pages to be colored. After reading through the names of the meridians, abbreviations, and assigned colors, start playing!

| Meridian | Abbreviation | Color |
|---|---|---|
| Lung | LU | Gray |
| Large Intestine | LI | White |
| Stomach | ST | Yellow |
| Spleen | SP | Violet |
| Heart | HE | Red |
| Small Intestine | SI | Orange |
| Bladder | BL | Light blue |
| Kidney | KI | Deep blue or indigo |
| Pericardium | PC | Silver |
| Triple Warmer | TW | Pink |
| Gallbladder | GB | Green |
| Liver | LR | Brown |
| Conception vessel or Ren Mai | CV | Black |
| Governor vessel | GV | Black |

## ILLUSTRATIONS OF THE MAJOR MERIDIANS

Feel free to select colors of your choice to color in the titles of the pages containing front and back views of all the main meridians. Once you get to the individual meridians, use the corresponding color from the instructions on the facing page.

*See pages 30–33 for the Major Meridians.*

## ILLUSTRATIONS OF INDIVIDUAL MERIDIANS

In the following pages, you will find that each English-language meridian name is followed by a Chinese term that further defines the nature of the meridian. This term contains either "yin" or "yang," followed by one of the four words in the following list.

| Term | Meaning | Color |
|------|---------|-------|
| Tai | Greater | Red |
| Ming | Brightness | Yellow |
| Shao | Lesser | Blue |
| Jue | Absolute | Gold |

You will be coloring the English and Chinese names on the instruction pages in this section.

## LUNG MERIDIAN: TAI YIN

This meridian begins at the Triple Warmer near the navel, runs inside the chest, and surfaces in front of the shoulder. Here it branches out from the armpits to run down the medial aspect of the upper arms and crosses at the crease of the elbows. It continues until it splits into two more branches, one flowing to the tips of the thumbs and the other to the ends of the index fingers. The branching is implied on the left side, which isn't shown on the figure. Another branch runs from the chest to the large intestine. This divergent channel is shown with dotted lines.

The lung regulates chi throughout the body as well as breathing and many water channels, such as the kidney and bladder. Symptoms of disharmony include distension of or a full sensation in the chest, asthma, allergies, coughing, panting, belching, restlessness, cold limbs and hot palms, shortness of breath, skin issues, and overall fatigue.

*See pages 34–35 for the Lung Meridian.*

## LARGE INTESTINE MERIDIAN: YANG MING

The Large Intestine meridian starts in the tip of each index finger and rises along the lateral side of the forearm and the anterior side of the upper arm to reach the highest points in the shoulder. Here it diverges into two branches. One travels internally into the lungs, diaphragm, and large intestine. The other flows externally, passing the neck and cheek to enter the lower teeth and gums, and then on to the end of the nose. The point extending into the forehead is officially Gallbladder-14 and can be used to work on the Large Intestine meridian.

The Large Intestine meridian rules elimination and communicates with the lungs to regulate the transportation functions of the body. This meridian primarily underlies diseases that affect the head, face, and throat. Disharmony is indicated by toothaches, runny noses, nosebleeds, swelling of the neck, yellow eyes, dry mouth, excessive thirst, sore throat, and pain in the shoulders, arms, and index fingers, as well as intestinal cramping, diarrhea, constipation, and dysentery.

*See pages 36–37 for the Large Intestine Meridian.*

## STOMACH MERIDIAN: YANG MING

The Stomach meridian emerges from the end of the Large Intestine meridian just under the eyes. It then goes around the nose to encircle the bridge of the nose, simultaneously going down around the mouth and up each cheek to the forehead. It then travels from the lower jaw through the neck to the sternum, where it divides into two branches. One branch passes down the chest, belly, and groin and continues down each leg, ending at the tip of the second toe.

The Stomach meridian works closely with the Spleen meridian to perform digestion and absorption. Together, the two meridians are called the acquired foundation; they lay the foundation of digestive health for the body. The Stomach meridian assures that the chi descends or is passed into the internal system. Diseases involving the Stomach meridian typically produce gastric disturbances, toothaches, and mental issues (such as obsessively going over the same thoughts), as well as problems associated with the meridian's path. Irregularities can appear as stomachaches, mouth sores, digestive disturbances, fluid in the abdomen, hunger, nausea, vomiting, thirst, a distorted mouth, edema, swollen neck, sore throat, shuddering, yawning, and a gray forehead. Mental dysfunctions include antisocial and phobic behavior.

*See pages 38–39 for the Stomach Meridian.*

## SPLEEN MERIDIAN: TAI YIN

The Spleen meridian starts at the big toe and moves along the inside of the foot, then turns at the inner ankle and climbs to the armpit. One branch leaves the abdomen and runs inside the body to the spleen, linking with the stomach and the heart.

The spleen is a vital immune organ and is essential for transforming food into chi and blood. It is also considered to house thoughts, governing the quality of thought available to the mind. Symptoms of related diseases include a distended abdomen, loss of appetite, hepatitis, bleeding disorders, menstrual disorders, loose stools, diarrhea, flatulence, anorexia, stiffness, swollen or stiff knees or thighs, and pain at the root of the tongue.

*See pages 40–41 for the Spleen Meridian.*

## HEART MERIDIAN: SHAO YIN

The Heart meridian starts in the heart and consists of three branches. One goes to the small intestine. Another runs upward past the tongue toward the eyes. The third branch crosses the chest to travel down the arm, ending at the inside top of the little finger, where it connects with the Small Intestine meridian.

The Heart meridian governs the blood and the pulse, as well as the mind and spirit. As might be expected, problems with the Heart meridian usually result in heart problems, which can be indicated by dry throat, heart pain, palpitations, and thirst. Other symptoms include pain in the chest or along the inner side of the forearm, heat in the palm, yellow eyes, insomnia, and pain or cold along the meridian pathway.

*See pages 42–43 for the Heart Meridian.*

## SMALL INTESTINE MERIDIAN: TAI YANG

The Small Intestine meridian begins in the outside tip of the little finger and goes up the arm to the back of the shoulder. At the intersection of the Bladder meridian, it diverges into two branches. One branch moves internally through the heart and stomach to settle in the small intestine. The other branch travels externally around the cheeks on the face, passing through the eye and ear. A short branch off the cheek links the meridian to the inner corner of the eye, where it connects with the Bladder meridian.

The Small Intestine meridian separates the pure from the impure, including foods, fluids, thoughts, and beliefs. Problems in the Small Intestine meridian usually create diseases of the neck, ears, eyes, throat, head, and small intestine, as well as certain mental illnesses. Symptoms can include fevers, sore throats, swollen chin or lower cheek, stiff neck, fixed head stance, hearing problems or deafness, yellow eyes, severe pain of the shoulder, lower jaw, upper arm, elbow, and forearm, and disorders including irritable bowel syndrome.

*See pages 44–45 for the Small Intestine Meridian.*

## BLADDER MERIDIAN: TAI YANG

The Bladder meridian begins its journey at the inside edge of each eye and travels over the top of the head (where it visits the brain) to the back of the neck. Here it splits in two parts. One (the inner branch) travels into the base of the neck and moves down parallel with the spine. At the bottom, it reaches into the bladder. The other branch moves across the back of the shoulder and then runs downward alongside the inner branch. The two branches move through the buttocks and join at the knees. Each meridian now continues down the back of the lower leg, circles the outer ankle, and finally ends at the tip of the little toe, where it connects with (but is not the start of) the Kidney meridian.

The Bladder meridian is in charge of storing and eliminating fluid waste. It receives chi from the Kidney meridian and uses it to transform fluids for eliminating. Dysfunction of the Bladder meridian leads to bladder problems and symptoms including urinary disorders, incontinence, and problems in the head including headaches, protruding eyeballs, runny nose, nasal congestion, neck tension, yellow eyes, tearing, and nosebleeds. Lower-body issues include pain along the spine, buttocks, and calf muscles, lumbar pain, unbendable hip joints, groin issues, and tight muscles around the knee and in the calves.

*See pages 46–47 for the Bladder Meridian.*

## KIDNEY MERIDIAN: SHAO YIN

The Kidney meridian initiates between the long bones of the second and third toes, near the sole of the foot. It travels the inside of the leg, entering the body near the base of the spine. At the kidneys, it splits into two branches. These pass through the chest and intersect at the Pericardium meridian, and from there journey to the base of the tongue. (A small branch divides at the lungs to link with the heart and the pericardium.)

According to classical sources, kidneys "grasp the chi." They are the "residence" of yin and yang. They also rule the bones, teeth, and adrenal glands. Lack of nourishment results in kidney-based problems such as swelling, diarrhea, and constipation. Other symptoms include backaches, ear problems, anorexia, restlessness, insomnia, weak vision, lack of energy, constant fear, dry tongue and hot mouth, spinal and thigh pain, immovable lower limbs, cold, drowsiness, and painful and hot soles of the feet.

*See pages 48–49 for the Kidney Meridian.*

## PERICARDIUM MERIDIAN: JUE YIN

The Pericardium meridian starts near the heart, where it divides into two branches. One emerges from the lower chest area to reach the armpit before reversing down the arm to end at the tip of the middle finger. The other branch takes the same path but stops at the ring finger, where it meets the Triple Warmer (this extended branch is not shown).

The Pericardium meridian works closely with the Heart meridian; in fact, the pericardium is a bag that contains the heart, protecting it from foreign invasions. This meridian governs the blood and the mind (along with the Heart meridian), thus affecting blood and circulation as well as personal relationships. Disharmony in the Pericardium meridian is caused by heart and blood dysfunctions. The most common problems manifest as chest, heart, and breast problems, with symptoms including chest discomfort, tachycardia or other arrhythmias, swelling in the armpit, red face, spasms of the elbow and arm, and mania.

Note that the heart stores *shen*, or mental energy. Many mental or emotional problems relate to an imbalance in shen. The Pericardium is an important meridian for any symptoms related to mental illness. There are specific shen points listed in classical and other acupuncture manuals.

*See pages 50–51 for the Pericardium Meridian.*

## TRIPLE WARMER MERIDIAN: SHAO YANG

The Triple Warmer is not represented by a physical organ. Rather, it is important because of its job, which is to circulate liquid energy throughout the organs. It begins at the tip of the ring finger and flows over the shoulder to the chest cavity. Atop the chest cavity, it splits into two branches. One branch travels through the middle and lower parts of the body, uniting the upper, middle, and lower burners (hence the name, Triple Warmer or Burner). The other runs externally up the side of the neck, circling the face to finally meet the Gallbladder meridian at the outer ends of the eyebrow.

The Triple Warmer distributes a special chi called source chi, which is produced by the kidneys. It governs the relationship between all the various organs, allocating chi between them. You will be coloring in the labels of the Triple Warmer using pink. You can mix it up and use different shades of pink for Upper, Middle, and Lower Warmers. Try rose, light pink, salmon, or hot pink, if you have them.

**Upper Warmer:** Distributes chi from the diaphragm upward; most commonly associated with lungs and heart (respiration).

**Middle Warmer:** Delivers chi to bodily areas between the diaphragm and navel; associated with stomach, spleen, liver, and gallbladder (digestion and assimilation).

**Lower Warmer:** Transports chi below the navel; associated with reproduction and elimination.

Problems with the Triple Warmer typically manifest as water retention, stiff neck, and ailments with the ears, eyes, chest, and throat. Symptoms include those related to water imbalance, such as swelling, urinary incontinence and difficulties, and tinnitus (ringing in the ear).

*See pages 52–53 for the Triple Warmer Meridian.*

## GALLBLADDER MERIDIAN: SHAO YANG

The Gallbladder meridian starts as two branches emerging from the outer corner of the eye. An external branch weaves around the face and ear before traveling to the hip. The other branch crosses the cheek and descends to the gallbladder to meet up with the external branch. This rejoined branch now runs down the lateral side of the thigh and lower leg and makes its way to the tip of the fourth toe. Another small branch separates from the meridian at this point and ends at the big toe, where it connects with the Liver meridian.

The Gallbladder meridian runs the gallbladder, which makes and stores bile. On an energetic basis, it governs decision making. It is closely connected to the liver; therefore, many symptoms display as liver issues, including bitterness in the mouth, jaundice, and nausea. Other symptoms include frequent sighing, headaches, pain in the jaw and outer corner of the eyes, swelling in the glands, mental illness, indecisiveness, fever, and pain along the meridian.

*See pages 54–55 for the Gallbladder Meridian.*

## LIVER MERIDIAN: JUE YIN

The Liver meridian starts at the top of the big toe and travels up the leg to the pubic bone. It then circles the sexual organs, enters the lower abdomen, and travels upward to connect with the liver and gallbladder. It moves up to the lungs to connect with the Lung meridian before curving around the mouth. It then splits, and one branch goes up to each eye. The two disjointed branches finally meet at the forehead and travel over the top of the head.

To some practitioners of Traditional Chinese Medicine, the liver is considered the "second heart" of the body, thus indicating its importance. This meridian assures the flow of emotions, chi, and blood, controls the body's immune response as well as sinews (tendons, ligaments, and skeletal muscles), absorbs what is indigestible, and is associated with the eyes. Liver meridian issues most frequently appear as problems in the liver and genital systems. Symptoms can include dizziness, high blood pressure, hernias,

distended lower abdomens in women, nausea, watery stools with undigested food, allergies, incontinence, muscle spasms, retention of urine, eye problems, and moodiness or anger.

*See pages 56–57 for the Liver Meridian.*

## CONCEPTION VESSEL: REN MAI

Like the Governor vessel, the Conception vessel distributes chi to the major organs and maintains the proper balance of chi and blood. The Conception vessel runs up the front of the body, from the perineum to just below the eyes. Problems with this vessel include uneasiness, hernias, and abdominal issues. It is yin in nature.

*See pages 58–59 for the Conception Vessel.*

## GOVERNOR VESSEL: DU MAI

Like the Conception vessel, the Governor vessel transports chi to the major organs and balances the chi and blood in the body. The Governor vessel starts at the perineum and travels to the coccyx before making its way to the back of the head. Flowing over the head, it then travels down the front of the face to stop at the canines in the upper jaw. Disharmony in this vessel can cause symptoms including stiffness and scoliosis. It is yang in nature.

*See pages 60–61 for the Governor Vessel.*

## HEAD MERIDIANS

Many of the meridians run through the head. The related acupoints are helpful for conditions ranging from headaches to insomnia and can benefit the entire body.

*See pages 62–63 for the Head Meridians.*

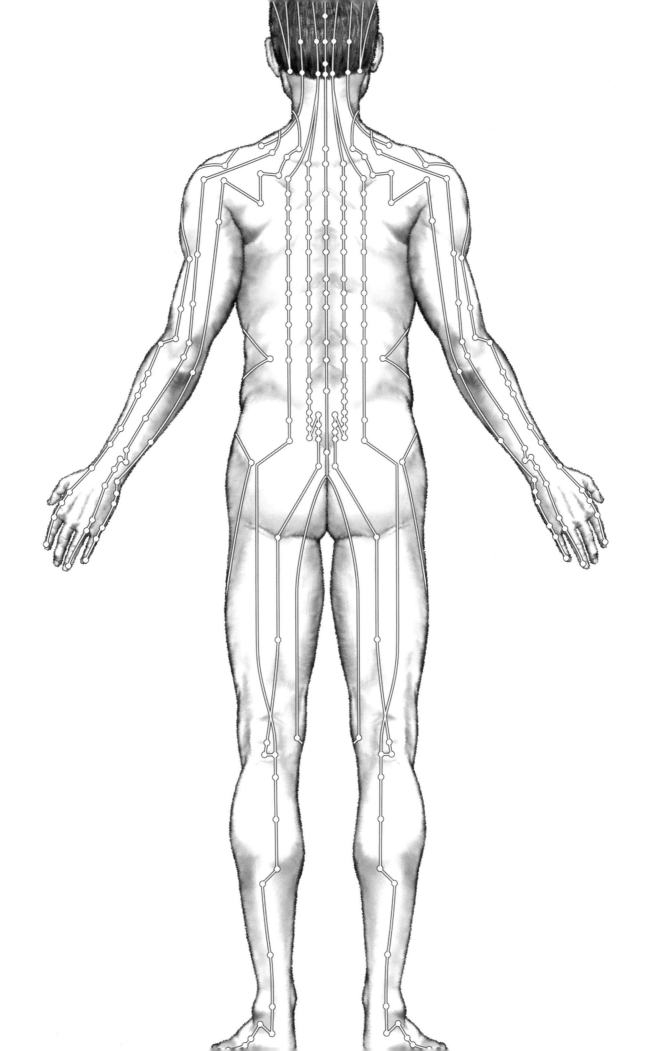

# MAJOR MERIDIANS: FRONT VIEW

Color in each meridian according to the suggested colors below, and write the abbreviation next to the labels using the same color.

BL     BLADDER MERIDIAN   light blue

CV     CONCEPTION VESSEL   black

ST     STOMACH MERIDIAN   yellow

LU     LUNG MERIDIAN   gray

KI     KIDNEY MERIDIAN   deep blue/indigo

LI     LARGE INTESTINE MERIDIAN   white

GB     GALLBLADDER MERIDIAN   green

HE     HEART MERIDIAN   red

LR     LIVER MERIDIAN   brown

PC     PERICARDIUM MERIDIAN   silver

SI     SMALL INTESTINE MERIDIAN   orange

SP     SPLEEN MERIDIAN   violet

TW     TRIPLE WARMER MERIDIAN   pink

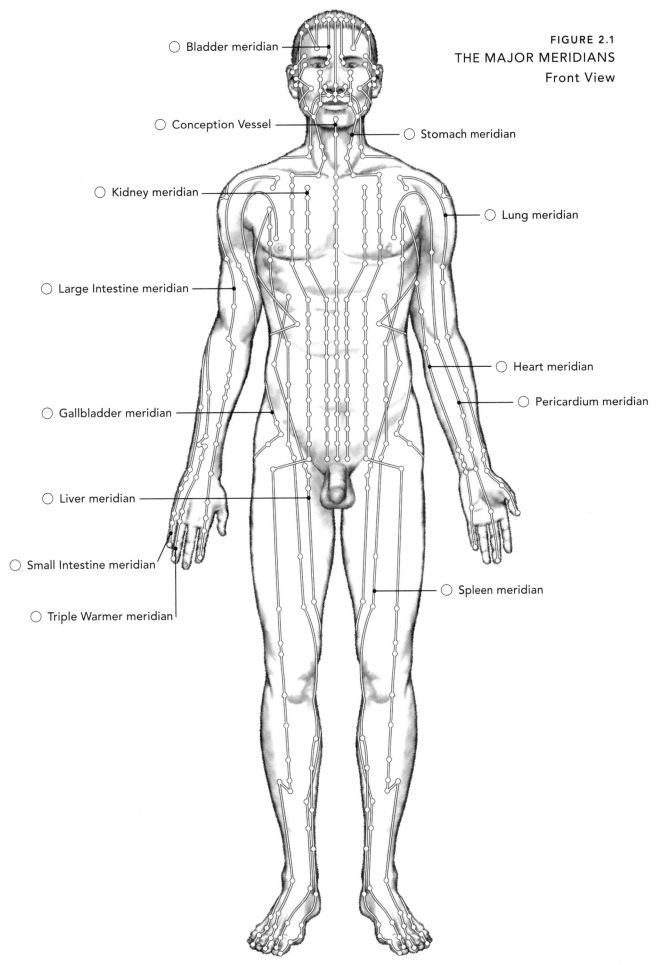

FIGURE 2.1
THE MAJOR MERIDIANS
Front View

○ Bladder meridian

○ Conception Vessel

○ Stomach meridian

○ Kidney meridian

○ Lung meridian

○ Large Intestine meridian

○ Heart meridian

○ Pericardium meridian

○ Gallbladder meridian

○ Liver meridian

○ Small Intestine meridian

○ Spleen meridian

○ Triple Warmer meridian

# MAJOR MERIDIANS: BACK VIEW

Color in each meridian according to the suggested colors below, and write the abbreviation next to the labels using the same color.

BL     BLADDER MERIDIAN   light blue

GV     GOVERNOR VESSEL   black

KI     KIDNEY MERIDIAN   deep blue/indigo

LI     LARGE INTESTINE MERIDIAN   white

GB     GALLBLADDER MERIDIAN   green

SI     SMALL INTESTINE MERIDIAN   orange

TW     TRIPLE WARMER MERIDIAN   pink

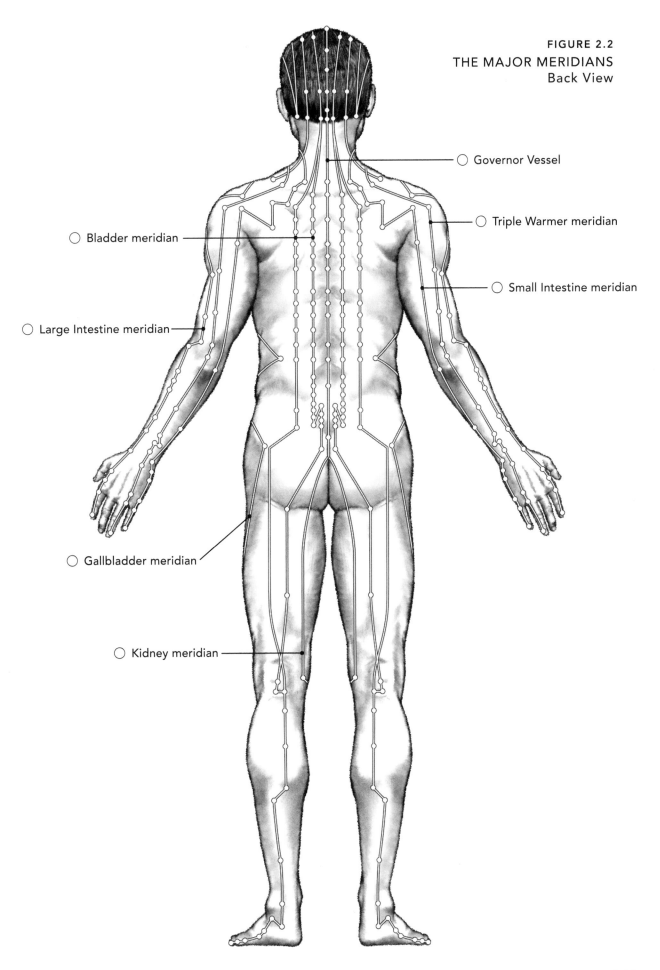

FIGURE 2.2
THE MAJOR MERIDIANS
Back View

○ Governor Vessel

○ Triple Warmer meridian

○ Bladder meridian

○ Small Intestine meridian

○ Large Intestine meridian

○ Gallbladder meridian

○ Kidney meridian

# LUNG MERIDIAN: LU gray

Color the main meridian and its English and Chinese labels with the color assigned to the meridian. Fill in the dotted or secondary lines with silver, trace the arrows with black, and fill in the acupoints with the indicated colors. If no color is suggested below, choose your own.

## MERIDIAN DETAILS

| | | |
|---|---|---|
| Yin/Yang | YIN | white |
| Quality | TAI | greater, red |
| Partner meridian | LARGE INTESTINE | yang, white |
| Polar opposite | BLADDER | light blue |
| Element | METAL | white |
| Body clock | 3 A.M. – 5 A.M. | yellow |
| Emotion | GRIEF | white |
| Season | AUTUMN | white |
| Flavor | SPICY | white |

## ACUPOINTS

| | | |
|---|---|---|
| LU-1 | ALARM POINT | red |
| LU-5 | HE-SEA | water, black |
| LU-6 | XI-CLEFT | pink |
| LU-7 | LUO-CONNECTING | violet |
| LU-8 | JING-RIVER | metal, yellow |
| LU-9 | SHU-STREAM | earth, Yuan-source, brown or light blue |
| LU-10 | YING-SPRING | fire, orange |
| LU-11 | JING-WELL | wood, gray |

**FIGURE 2.3**
LUNG MERIDIAN
Tai Yin

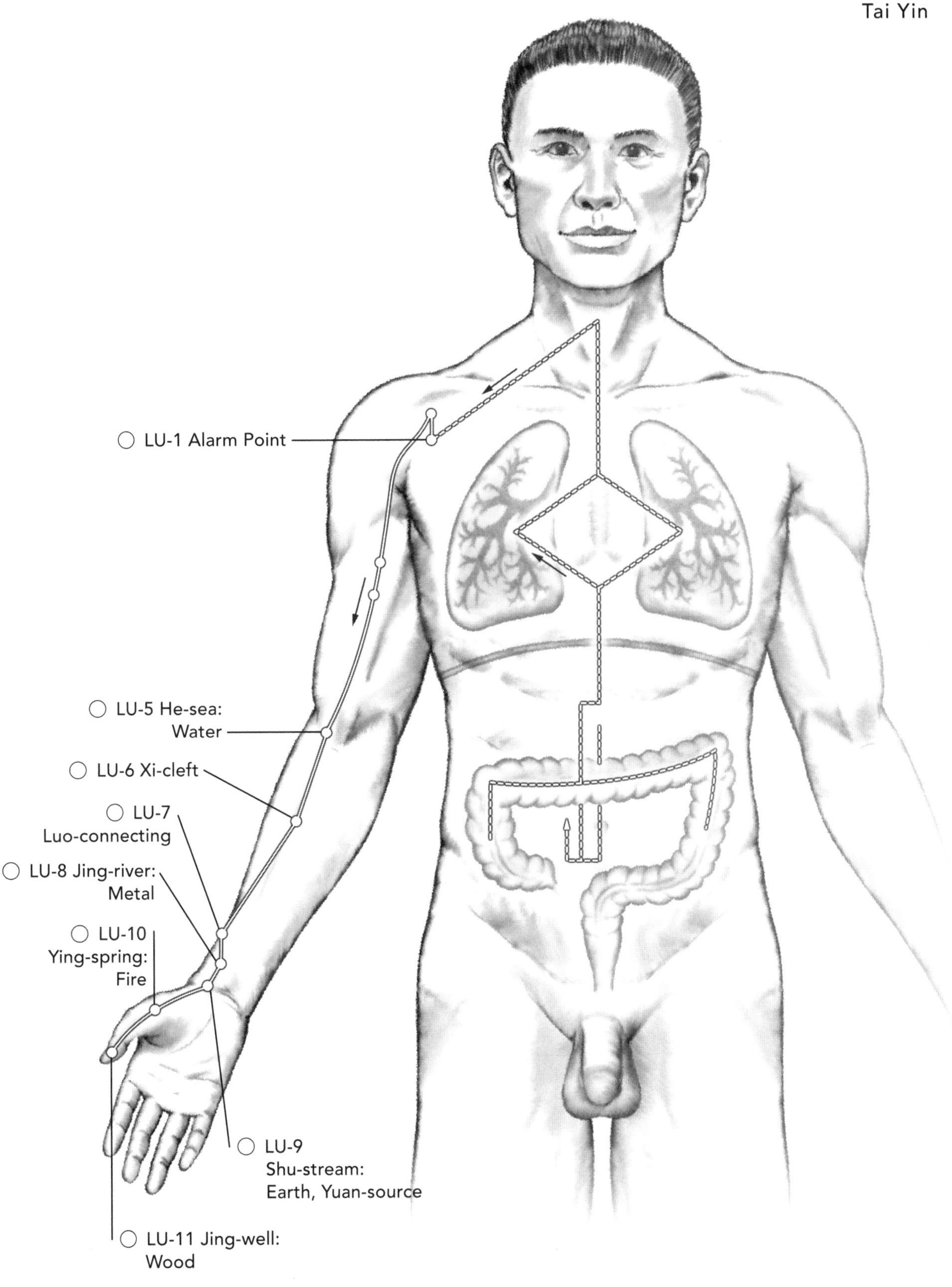

○ LU-1 Alarm Point

○ LU-5 He-sea:
Water

○ LU-6 Xi-cleft

○ LU-7
Luo-connecting

○ LU-8 Jing-river:
Metal

○ LU-10
Ying-spring:
Fire

○ LU-9
Shu-stream:
Earth, Yuan-source

○ LU-11 Jing-well:
Wood

# LARGE INTESTINE MERIDIAN: LI white

Color the main meridian and its English and Chinese labels with the color assigned to the meridian. Fill in the dotted or secondary lines with silver, trace the arrows with black, and fill in the acupoints with the indicated colors. If no color is suggested below, choose your own.

## MERIDIAN DETAILS

| | | |
|---|---|---|
| Yin/Yang | YANG | black |
| Quality | MING | brightness, yellow |
| Partner meridian | LUNG | gray |
| Polar opposite | KIDNEY | deep blue/indigo |
| Element | METAL | white |
| Body clock | 5 A.M. – 7 A.M. | yellow |
| Emotion | GRIEF | white |
| Season | AUTUMN | white |
| Flavor | SPICY | white |

## ACUPOINTS

| | | |
|---|---|---|
| LI-1 | JING-WELL | metal, gray |
| LI-2 | YING-SPRING | water, orange |
| LI-3 | SHU-STREAM | wood, brown |
| LI-4 | YUAN-SOURCE | light blue |
| LI-5 | JING-RIVER | fire, yellow |
| LI-6 | LUO-CONNECTING | violet |
| LI-7 | XI-CLEFT | pink |
| LI-11 | HE-SEA | earth, black |

**FIGURE 2.4**
LARGE INTESTINE MERIDIAN
Yang Ming

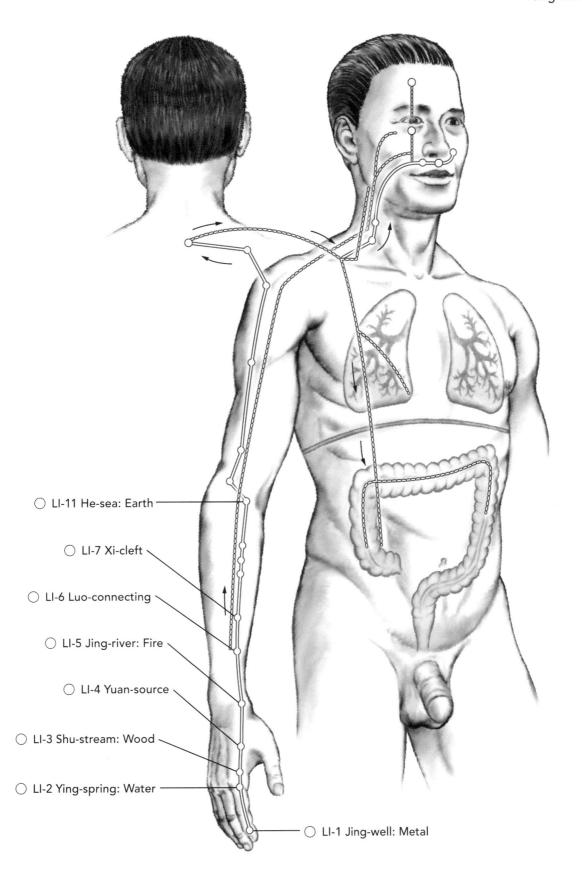

○ LI-11 He-sea: Earth

○ LI-7 Xi-cleft

○ LI-6 Luo-connecting

○ LI-5 Jing-river: Fire

○ LI-4 Yuan-source

○ LI-3 Shu-stream: Wood

○ LI-2 Ying-spring: Water

○ LI-1 Jing-well: Metal

# STOMACH MERIDIAN: ST yellow

Color the main meridian and its English and Chinese labels with the color assigned to the meridian. Fill in the dotted or secondary lines with silver, trace the arrows with black, and fill in the acupoints with the indicated colors. If no color is suggested below, choose your own.

## MERIDIAN DETAILS

| | | |
|---|---|---|
| Yin/Yang | YANG | black |
| Quality | MING | brightness, yellow |
| Partner meridian | SPLEEN | violet |
| Polar opposite | PERICARDIUM | silver |
| Element | EARTH | yellow |
| Body clock | 7 A.M. - 9 A.M. | yellow |
| Emotion | OVERTHINKING | yellow |
| Season | LATE SUMMER | yellow |
| Flavor | SWEET | yellow |

## ACUPOINTS

| | | |
|---|---|---|
| ST-34 | XI-CLEFT | pink |
| ST-36 | HE-SEA | earth, black |
| ST-40 | LUO-CONNECTING | violet |
| ST-41 | JING-RIVER | fire, yellow |
| ST-42 | YUAN-SOURCE | light blue |
| ST-43 | SHU-STREAM | wood, brown |
| ST-44 | YING-SPRING | water, orange |
| ST-45 | JING-WELL | metal, gray |

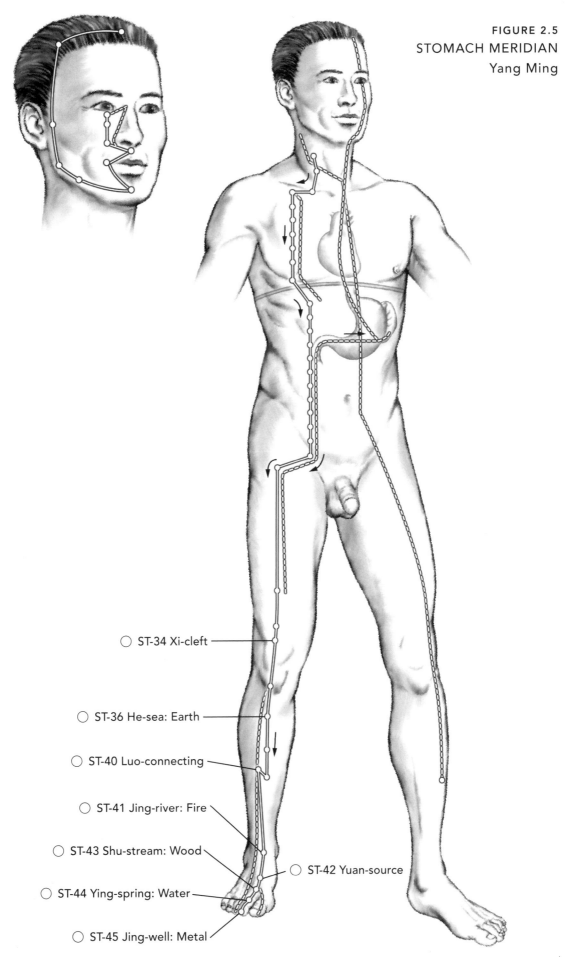

FIGURE 2.5
STOMACH MERIDIAN
Yang Ming

○ ST-34 Xi-cleft

○ ST-36 He-sea: Earth

○ ST-40 Luo-connecting

○ ST-41 Jing-river: Fire

○ ST-43 Shu-stream: Wood

○ ST-42 Yuan-source

○ ST-44 Ying-spring: Water

○ ST-45 Jing-well: Metal

# SPLEEN MERIDIAN: SP <sub>violet</sub>

Color the main meridian and its English and Chinese labels with the color assigned to the meridian. Fill in the dotted or secondary lines with silver, trace the arrows with black, and fill in the acupoints with the indicated colors. If no color is suggested below, choose your own.

## MERIDIAN DETAILS

| | | |
|---|---|---|
| Yin/Yang | YIN | white |
| Quality | TAI | greater, red |
| Partner meridian | STOMACH | yang, yellow |
| Polar opposite | TRIPLE WARMER | pink |
| Element | EARTH | yellow |
| Body clock | 9 A.M. – 11 A.M. | yellow |
| Emotion | OVERTHINKING | yellow |
| Season | LATE SUMMER | yellow |
| Flavor | SWEET | yellow |

## ACUPOINTS

| | | |
|---|---|---|
| SP-1 | JING-WELL | wood, gray |
| SP-2 | YING-SPRING | fire, orange |
| SP-3 | SHU-STREAM | earth, Yuan-source, brown or light blue |
| SP-4 | LUO-CONNECTING | violet |
| SP-5 | JING-RIVER | metal, yellow |
| SP-8 | XI-CLEFT | pink |
| SP-9 | HE-SEA | water, black |

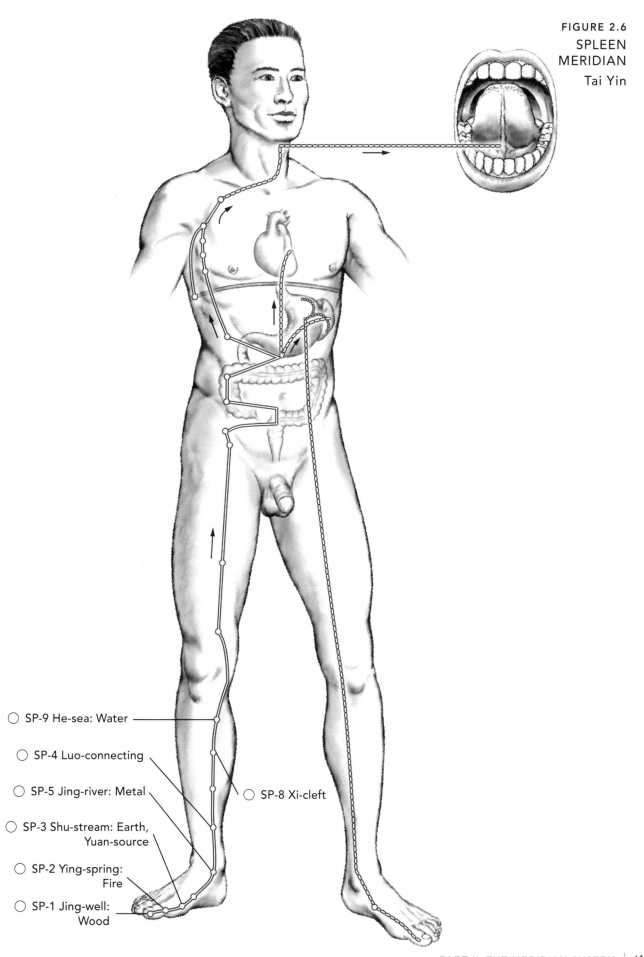

FIGURE 2.6
SPLEEN
MERIDIAN
Tai Yin

○ SP-9 He-sea: Water

○ SP-4 Luo-connecting

○ SP-5 Jing-river: Metal

○ SP-8 Xi-cleft

○ SP-3 Shu-stream: Earth,
Yuan-source

○ SP-2 Ying-spring:
Fire

○ SP-1 Jing-well:
Wood

# HEART MERIDIAN: HE <sub></sub> red

Color the main meridian and its English and Chinese labels with the color assigned to the meridian. Fill in the dotted or secondary lines with silver, trace the arrows with black, and fill in the acupoints with the indicated colors. If no color is suggested below, choose your own.

## MERIDIAN DETAILS

| | | |
|---|---|---|
| Yin/Yang | YIN | white |
| Quality | SHAO | lesser, blue |
| Partner meridian | SMALL INTESTINE | yang, orange |
| Polar opposite | GALLBLADDER | green |
| Element | FIRE | red |
| Body clock | 11 A.M. – 1 P.M. | yellow and blue |
| Emotion | JOY | red |
| Season | SUMMER | red |
| Flavor | BITTER | red |

## ACUPOINTS

| | | |
|---|---|---|
| HE-3 | HE-SEA | water, black |
| HE-4 | JING-RIVER | metal, yellow |
| HE-5 | LUO-CONNECTING | violet |
| HE-6 | XI-CLEFT | pink |
| HE-7 | SHU-STREAM | earth, Yuan-source, brown or light blue |
| HE-8 | YING-SPRING | fire, orange |
| HE-9 | JING-WELL | wood, gray |

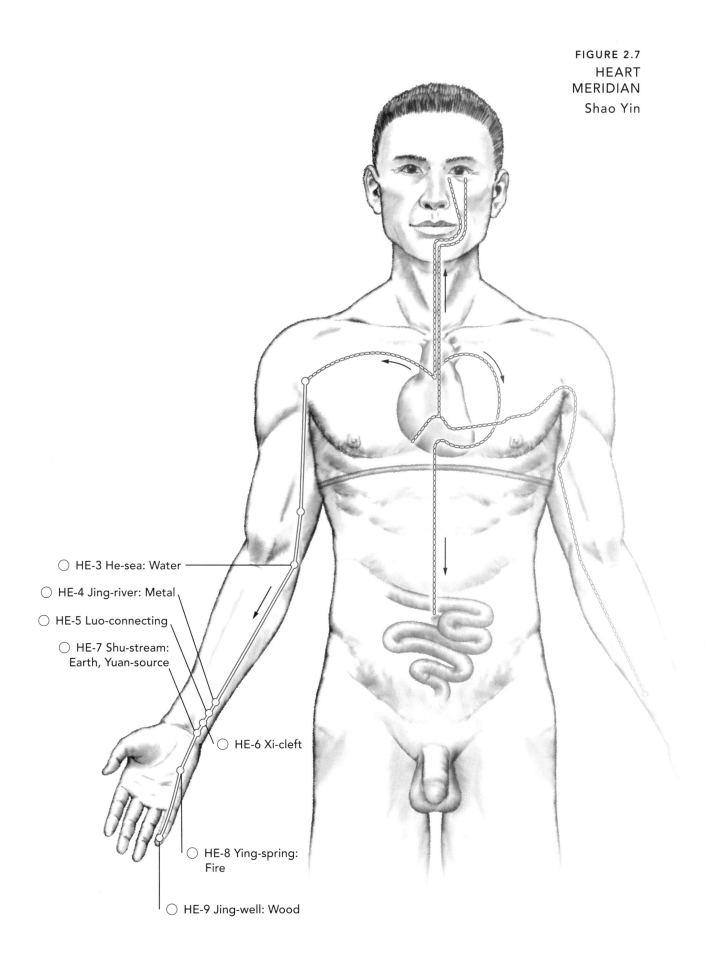

FIGURE 2.7
HEART
MERIDIAN
Shao Yin

○ HE-3 He-sea: Water

○ HE-4 Jing-river: Metal

○ HE-5 Luo-connecting

○ HE-7 Shu-stream:
Earth, Yuan-source

○ HE-6 Xi-cleft

○ HE-8 Ying-spring:
Fire

○ HE-9 Jing-well: Wood

# SMALL INTESTINE MERIDIAN: SI <small>orange</small>

Color the main meridian and its English and Chinese labels with the color assigned to the meridian. Fill in the dotted or secondary lines with silver, trace the arrows with black, and fill in the acupoints with the indicated colors. If no color is suggested below, choose your own.

## MERIDIAN DETAILS

| | | |
|---|---|---|
| Yin/Yang | YANG | black |
| Quality | TAI | greater, red |
| Partner meridian | HEART | red |
| Polar opposite | LIVER | brown |
| Element | FIRE | red |
| Body clock | 1 P.M. – 3 P.M. | blue |
| Emotion | JOY | red |
| Season | SUMMER | red |
| Flavor | BITTER | red |

## ACUPOINTS

| | | |
|---|---|---|
| SI-1 | JING-WELL | metal, gray |
| SI-2 | YING-SPRING | water, orange |
| SI-3 | SHU-STREAM | wood, brown |
| SI-4 | YUAN-SOURCE | light blue |
| SI-5 | JING-RIVER | fire, yellow |
| SI-6 | XI-CLEFT | pink |
| SI-7 | LUO-CONNECTING | violet |
| SI-8 | HE-SEA | earth, black |

FIGURE 2.8
SMALL INTESTINE
MERIDIAN
Tai Yang

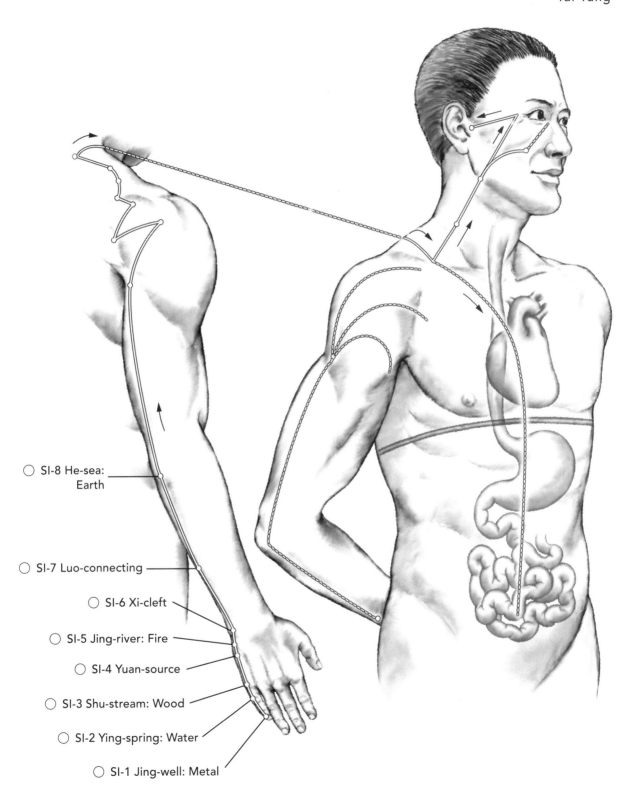

○ SI-8 He-sea:
   Earth

○ SI-7 Luo-connecting

○ SI-6 Xi-cleft

○ SI-5 Jing-river: Fire

○ SI-4 Yuan-source

○ SI-3 Shu-stream: Wood

○ SI-2 Ying-spring: Water

○ SI-1 Jing-well: Metal

# BLADDER MERIDIAN: BL light blue

Color the main meridian and its English and Chinese labels with the color assigned to the meridian. Fill in the dotted or secondary lines with silver, trace the arrows with black, and fill in the acupoints with the indicated colors. If no color is suggested below, choose your own.

## MERIDIAN DETAILS

| | | |
|---|---|---|
| Yin/Yang | YANG | black |
| Quality | TAI | greater, red |
| Partner meridian | KIDNEY | yin, deep blue/indigo |
| Polar opposite | LUNG | gray |
| Element | WATER | blue |
| Body clock | 3 P.M. – 5 P.M. | blue |
| Emotion | FEAR | blue |
| Season | WINTER | blue |
| Flavor | SALTY | blue |

## ASSOCIATED POINTS medium blue unless indicated

BL-13 LUNG

BL-14 PERICARDIUM

BL-15 HEART

BL-18 LIVER

BL-19 GALLBLADDER

BL-20 SPLEEN

BL-21 STOMACH

BL-22 TRIPLE WARMER

BL-23 KIDNEY

BL-25 LARGE INTESTINE

BL-27 SMALL INTESTINE

BL-28 BLADDER

## ACUPOINTS

BL-40 HE-SEA
earth, indigo or black

BL-58 LUO-CONNECTING
blue or violet

BL-60 JING-RIVER
fire, medium blue or yellow

BL-63 XI-CLEFT
medium blue or pink

BL-64 YUAN-SOURCE
light blue

BL-65 SHU-STREAM
wood, brown

BL-66 YING-SPRING
water, orange

BL-67 JING-WELL
metal, gray

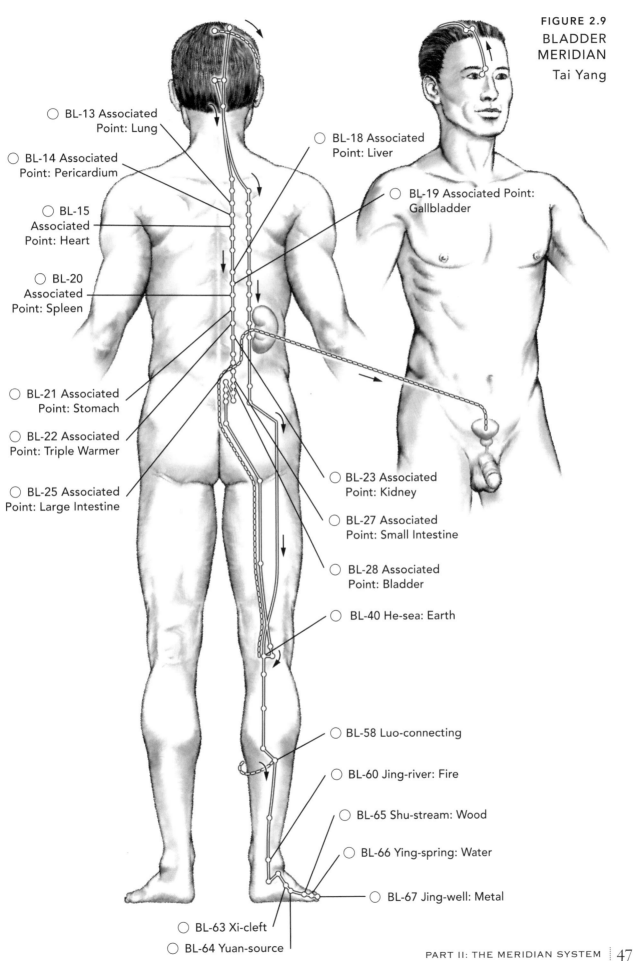

FIGURE 2.9
BLADDER
MERIDIAN
Tai Yang

○ BL-13 Associated
Point: Lung

○ BL-14 Associated
Point: Pericardium

○ BL-15
Associated
Point: Heart

○ BL-20
Associated
Point: Spleen

○ BL-21 Associated
Point: Stomach

○ BL-22 Associated
Point: Triple Warmer

○ BL-25 Associated
Point: Large Intestine

○ BL-18 Associated
Point: Liver

○ BL-19 Associated Point:
Gallbladder

○ BL-23 Associated
Point: Kidney

○ BL-27 Associated
Point: Small Intestine

○ BL-28 Associated
Point: Bladder

○ BL-40 He-sea: Earth

○ BL-58 Luo-connecting

○ BL-60 Jing-river: Fire

○ BL-65 Shu-stream: Wood

○ BL-66 Ying-spring: Water

○ BL-67 Jing-well: Metal

○ BL-63 Xi-cleft

○ BL-64 Yuan-source

# KIDNEY MERIDIAN: KI deep blue/indigo

Color the main meridian and its English and Chinese labels with the color assigned to the meridian. Fill in the dotted or secondary lines with silver, trace the arrows with black, and fill in the acupoints with the indicated colors. If no color is suggested below, choose your own.

## MERIDIAN DETAILS

| | | |
|---|---|---|
| Yin/Yang | YIN | white |
| Quality | SHAO | lesser, blue |
| Partner meridian | BLADDER | yang, light blue |
| Polar opposite | LARGE INTESTINE | white |
| Element | WATER | blue |
| Body clock | 5 P.M. – 7 P.M. | blue |
| Emotion | FEAR | blue |
| Season | WINTER | blue |
| Flavor | SALTY | blue |

## ACUPOINTS

| | | |
|---|---|---|
| KI-1 | JING-WELL | wood, gray |
| KI-2 | YING-SPRING | fire, orange |
| KI-3 | SHU-STREAM | earth, Yuan-source, brown or light blue |
| KI-4 | LUO-CONNECTING | violet |
| KI-5 | XI-CLEFT | pink |
| KI-7 | JING-RIVER | metal, yellow |
| KI-10 | HE-SEA | water, black |

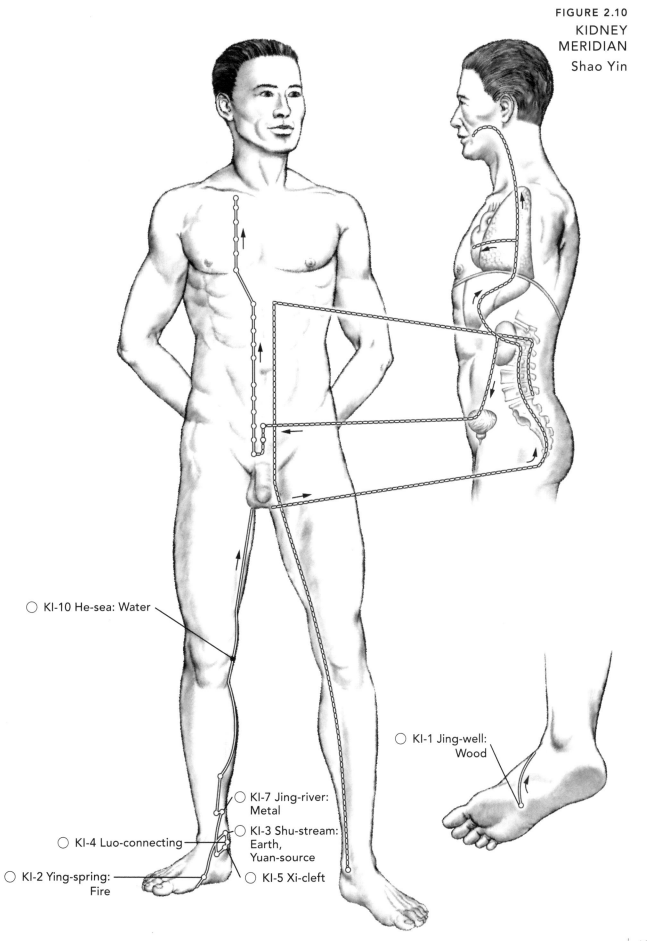

FIGURE 2.10
KIDNEY
MERIDIAN
Shao Yin

○ KI-10 He-sea: Water

○ KI-1 Jing-well: Wood

○ KI-7 Jing-river: Metal

○ KI-4 Luo-connecting

○ KI-3 Shu-stream: Earth, Yuan-source

○ KI-2 Ying-spring: Fire

○ KI-5 Xi-cleft

# PERICARDIUM MERIDIAN: PC silver

Color the main meridian and its English and Chinese labels with the color assigned to the meridian. Fill in the dotted or secondary lines with silver, trace the arrows with black, and fill in the acupoints with the indicated colors. If no color is suggested below, choose your own.

## MERIDIAN DETAILS

| | | |
|---|---|---|
| Yin/Yang | YIN | white |
| Quality | JUE | absolute, gold |
| Partner meridian | TRIPLE WARMER | pink |
| Polar opposite | STOMACH | yellow |
| Element | FIRE | red |
| Body clock | 7 P.M. – 9 P.M. | blue |
| Emotion | JOY | red |
| Season | SUMMER | red |
| Flavor | BITTER | red |

## ACUPOINTS

| | | |
|---|---|---|
| PC-3 | HE-SEA | water, black |
| PC-4 | XI-CLEFT | pink |
| PC-5 | JING-RIVER | metal, yellow |
| PC-6 | LUO-CONNECTING | violet |
| PC-7 | SHU-STREAM | earth, Yuan-source, brown or light blue |
| PC-8 | YING-SPRING | fire, orange |
| PC-9 | JING-WELL | wood, gray |

FIGURE 2.11

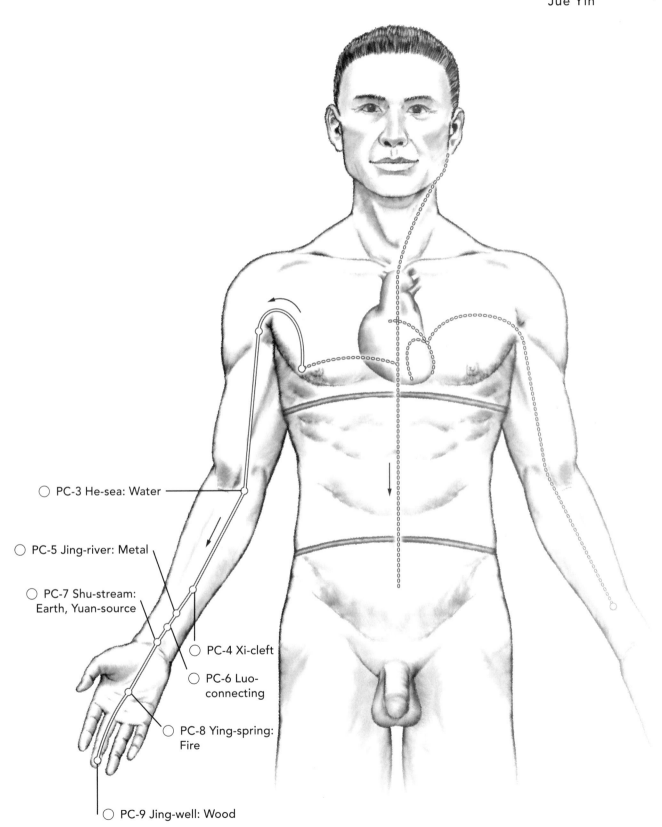

○ PC-3 He-sea: Water

○ PC-5 Jing-river: Metal

○ PC-7 Shu-stream:
Earth, Yuan-source

○ PC-4 Xi-cleft

○ PC-6 Luo-
connecting

○ PC-8 Ying-spring:
Fire

○ PC-9 Jing-well: Wood

# TRIPLE WARMER MERIDIAN: TW   pink

Color the main meridian and its English and Chinese labels with the color assigned to the meridian. Fill in the dotted or secondary lines with silver, trace the arrows with black, and fill in the acupoints with the indicated colors. If no color is suggested below, choose your own.

## MERIDIAN DETAILS

| | | |
|---|---|---|
| Yin/yang | YANG | black |
| Quality | SHAO | lesser, blue |
| Partner meridian | PERICARDIUM | silver |
| Polar opposite | SPLEEN | violet |
| Element | FIRE | red |
| Body clock | 9 P.M. – 11 P.M. | blue |
| Emotion | JOY | red |
| Season | SUMMER | red |
| Flavor | BITTER | red |

## ACUPOINTS

| | | |
|---|---|---|
| TW-1 | JING-WELL | metal, gray |
| TW-2 | YING-SPRING | water, orange |
| TW-3 | SHU-STREAM | wood, brown |
| TW-4 | YUAN-SOURCE | light blue |
| TW-5 | LUO-CONNECTING | violet |
| TW-6 | JING-RIVER | fire, yellow |
| TW-7 | XI-CLEFT | pink |
| TW-10 | HE-SEA | earth, black |

**FIGURE 2.12**
TRIPLE WARMER MERIDIAN
Shao Yang

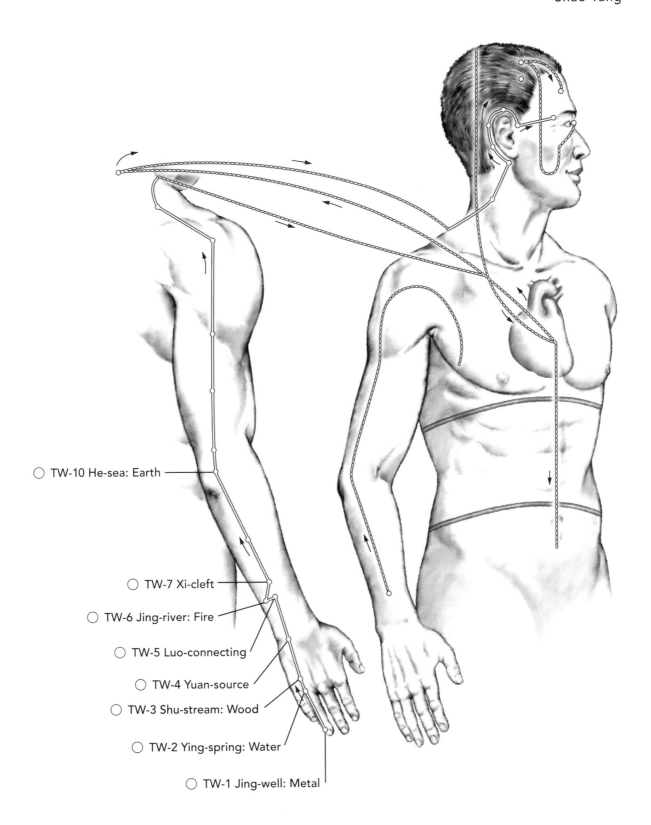

○ TW-10 He-sea: Earth

○ TW-7 Xi-cleft

○ TW-6 Jing-river: Fire

○ TW-5 Luo-connecting

○ TW-4 Yuan-source

○ TW-3 Shu-stream: Wood

○ TW-2 Ying-spring: Water

○ TW-1 Jing-well: Metal

# GALLBLADDER MERIDIAN: GB green

Color the main meridian and its English and Chinese labels with the color assigned to the meridian. Fill in the dotted or secondary lines with silver, trace the arrows with black, and fill in the acupoints with the indicated colors. If no color is suggested below, choose your own.

## MERIDIAN DETAILS

| | | |
|---|---|---|
| Yin/Yang | YANG | black |
| Quality | SHAO | lesser, blue |
| Partner meridian | LIVER | brown |
| Polar opposite | HEART | red |
| Element | WOOD | green |
| Body clock | 11 P.M. – 1 A.M. | yellow and blue |
| Emotion | ANGER | green |
| Season | SPRING | green |
| Flavor | SOUR | green |

## ACUPOINTS

GB-24    ALARM POINT red
GB-34    HE-SEA earth, black
GB-36    XI-CLEFT pink
GB-37    LUO-CONNECTING violet
GB-38    JING-RIVER fire, yellow
GB-40    YUAN-SOURCE light blue
GB-41    SHU-STREAM wood, brown
GB-43    YING-SPRING water, orange
GB-44    JING-WELL metal, gray

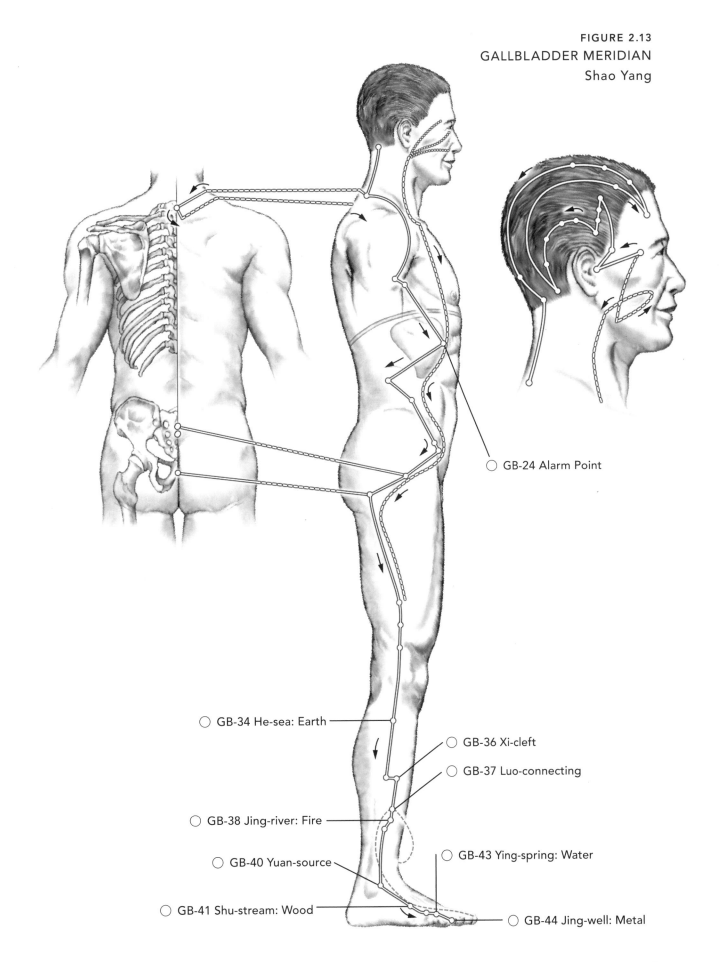

FIGURE 2.13
GALLBLADDER MERIDIAN
Shao Yang

○ GB-24 Alarm Point

○ GB-34 He-sea: Earth

○ GB-36 Xi-cleft

○ GB-37 Luo-connecting

○ GB-38 Jing-river: Fire

○ GB-43 Ying-spring: Water

○ GB-40 Yuan-source

○ GB-41 Shu-stream: Wood

○ GB-44 Jing-well: Metal

# LIVER MERIDIAN: LR brown

Color the main meridian and its English and Chinese labels with the color assigned to the meridian. Fill in the dotted or secondary lines with silver, trace the arrows with black, and fill in the acupoints with the indicated colors. If no color is suggested below, choose your own.

## MERIDIAN DETAILS

Yin/Yang            YIN white

Quality             JUE absolute, gold

Partner meridian    GALLBLADDER green

Polar opposite      SMALL INTESTINE orange

Element             WOOD green

Body clock          1 A.M. – 3 A.M. yellow

Emotion             ANGER green

Season              SPRING green

Flavor              SOUR green

## ACUPOINTS

LR-1    SHU-STREAM wood, brown

LR-2    JING-RIVER fire, yellow

LR-3    HE-SEA earth, Yuan-source, black or light blue

LR-4    JING-WELL metal, gray

LR-5    LUO-CONNECTING violet

LR-6    XI-CLEFT pink

LR-8    YING-SPRING water, orange

LR-14   ALARM POINT red

**FIGURE 2.14**
LIVER MERIDIAN
Jue Yin

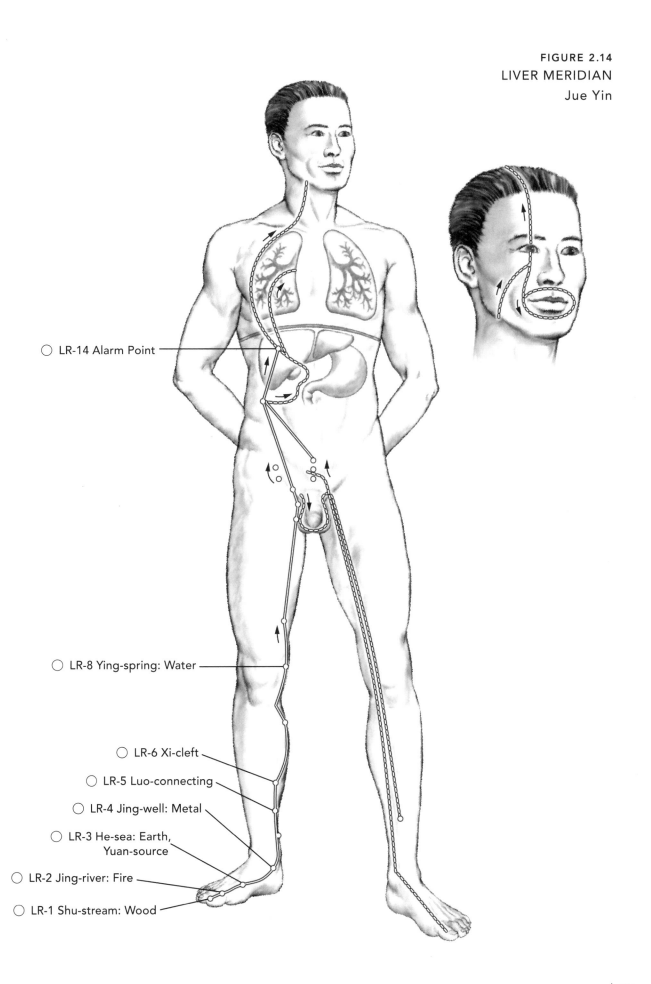

○ LR-14 Alarm Point

○ LR-8 Ying-spring: Water

○ LR-6 Xi-cleft

○ LR-5 Luo-connecting

○ LR-4 Jing-well: Metal

○ LR-3 He-sea: Earth,
   Yuan-source

○ LR-2 Jing-river: Fire

○ LR-1 Shu-stream: Wood

# CONCEPTION VESSEL: CV black

Color the main meridian and its English and Chinese labels with the color assigned to the meridian. Fill in the dotted or secondary lines with silver, trace the arrows with black, and fill in the acupoints with the indicated colors. If no color is suggested below, choose your own.

**ACUPOINTS**

CV-3     ALARM POINT
          BLADDER MERIDIAN   red

CV-4     ALARM POINT
          SMALL INTESTINE MERIDIAN   red

CV-5     ALARM POINT
          TRIPLE WARMER MERIDIAN   red

CV-5     CARDINAL POINT
          ENDOCRINE SYSTEM   red

CV-6     CARDINAL POINT
          LOWER ABDOMEN, SEXUAL ORGANS   silver

CV-12     ALARM POINT
          STOMACH MERIDIAN   red

CV-12     CARDINAL POINT
          UPPER ABDOMEN, YANG ORGANS   silver

CV-14     ALARM POINT
          HEART MERIDIAN   red

CV-15     LUO-CONNECTING   violet

CV-17     ALARM POINT
          PERICARDIUM MERIDIAN   red

CV-17     CARDINAL POINT
          CHEST, CENTER OF RESPIRATION   silver

FIGURE 2.15
CONCEPTION VESSEL
Ren Mai

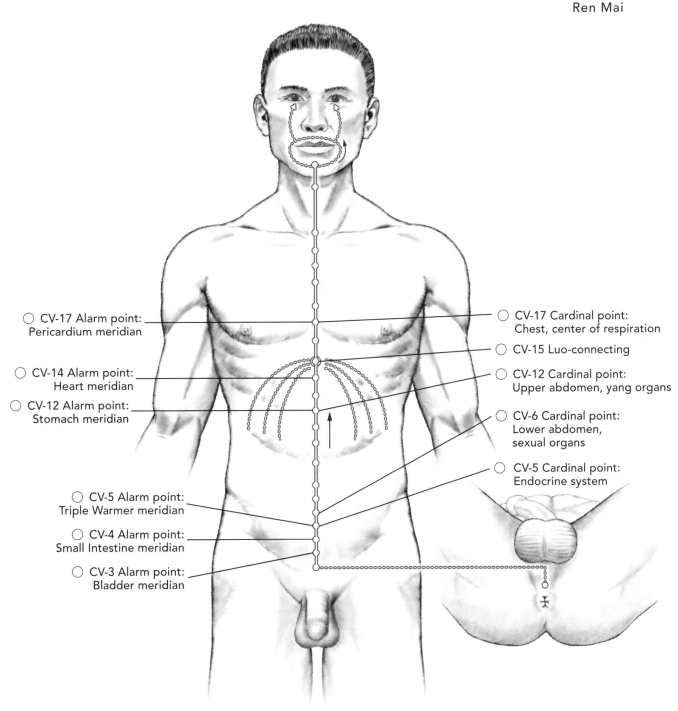

CV-17 Alarm point:
Pericardium meridian

CV-14 Alarm point:
Heart meridian

CV-12 Alarm point:
Stomach meridian

CV-5 Alarm point:
Triple Warmer meridian

CV-4 Alarm point:
Small Intestine meridian

CV-3 Alarm point:
Bladder meridian

CV-17 Cardinal point:
Chest, center of respiration

CV-15 Luo-connecting

CV-12 Cardinal point:
Upper abdomen, yang organs

CV-6 Cardinal point:
Lower abdomen,
sexual organs

CV-5 Cardinal point:
Endocrine system

# GOVERNOR VESSEL: CV black

Color the main meridian and its English and Chinese labels with the color assigned to the meridian. Fill in the dotted or secondary lines with silver, trace the arrows with black, and fill in the acupoints with the indicated colors. If no color is suggested below, choose your own.

## ACUPOINTS

GV-1    LUO-CONNECTING violet

GV-4    CARDINAL POINT
        IMMUNE SYSTEM silver

GV-14   CARDINAL POINT
        GENERAL (EXCESS ENERGY) silver

GV-20   CARDINAL POINT
        SKIN, SYMPATHETIC NERVOUS
        SYSTEM, MEMORY, MENTAL
        AND CEREBRAL DISORDERS silver

GV-26   CARDINAL POINT
        UNCONSCIOUSNESS,
        OBESITY silver

FIGURE 2.16
GOVERNOR VESSEL
Du Mai

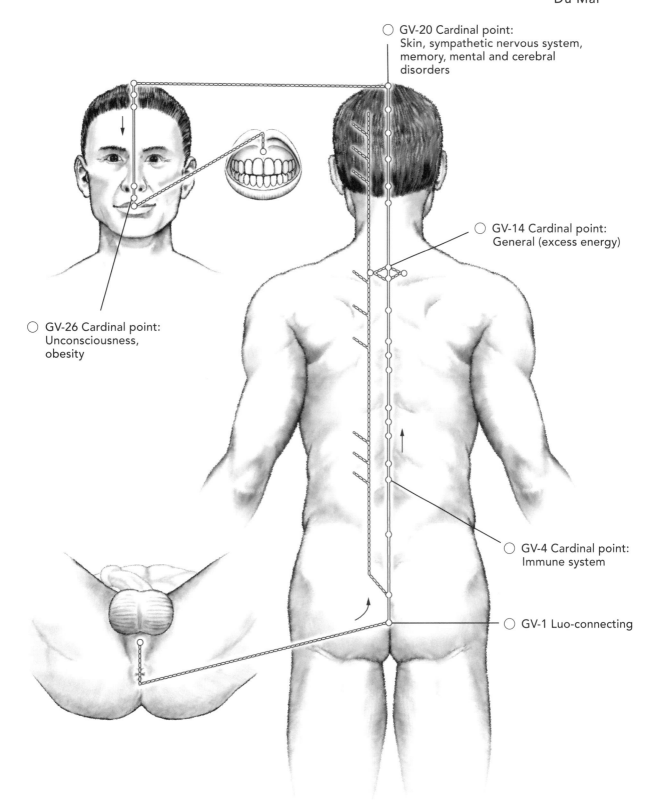

GV-20 Cardinal point:
Skin, sympathetic nervous system, memory, mental and cerebral disorders

GV-14 Cardinal point:
General (excess energy)

GV-26 Cardinal point:
Unconsciousness, obesity

GV-4 Cardinal point:
Immune system

GV-1 Luo-connecting

# HEAD MERIDIANS

Color the main meridian and its English and Chinese labels with the color assigned to the meridian. Fill in the dotted or secondary lines with silver, trace the arrows with black, and fill in the acupoints with the indicated colors. If no color is suggested below, choose your own.

GV     GOVERNOR VESSEL   black

BL     BLADDER MERIDIAN   light blue

GB     GALLBLADDER MERIDIAN   green

TW     TRIPLE WARMER MERIDIAN   pink

SI     SMALL INTESTINE MERIDIAN   orange

LI     LARGE INTESTINE MERIDIAN   white

ST     STOMACH MERIDIAN   yellow

FIGURE 2.17
HEAD MERIDIANS

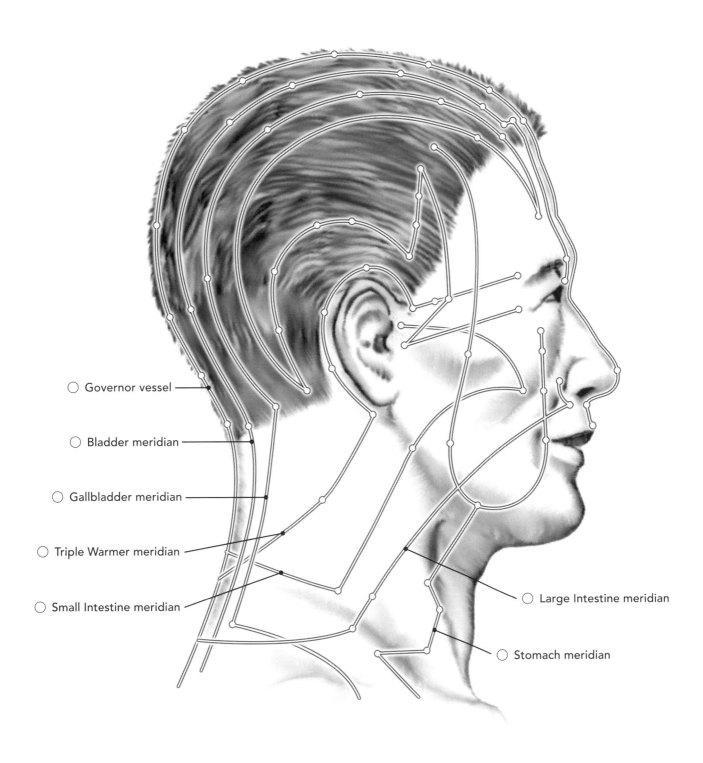

○ Governor vessel

○ Bladder meridian

○ Gallbladder meridian

○ Triple Warmer meridian

○ Small Intestine meridian

○ Large Intestine meridian

○ Stomach meridian

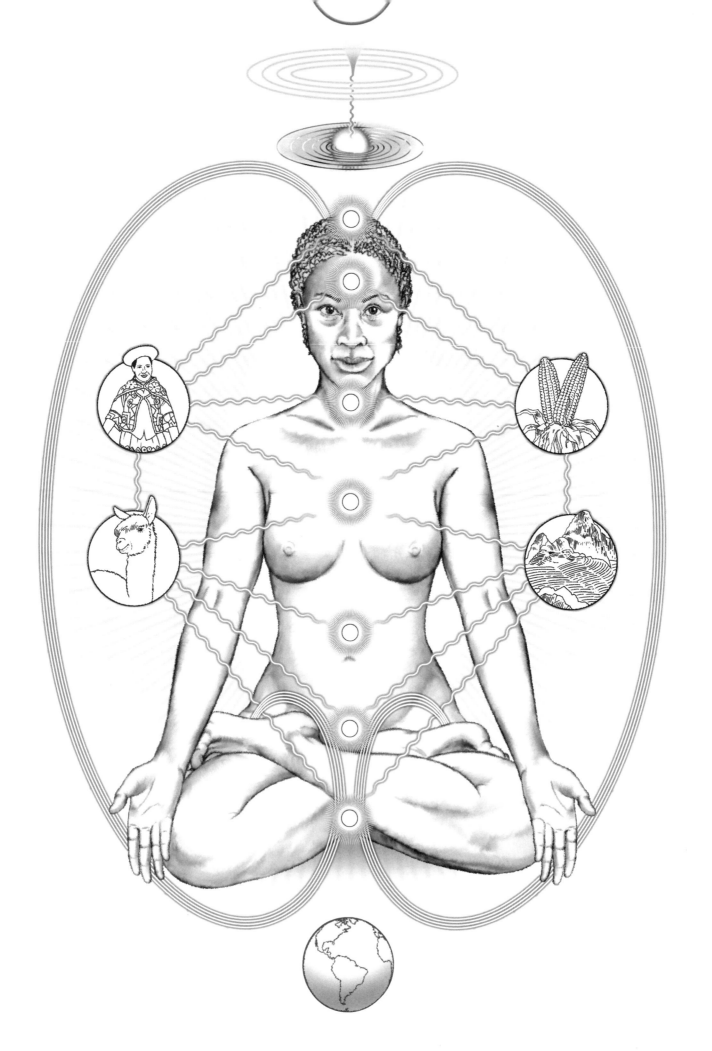

# PART III
## CHARKAS: ENERGY BODIES OF LIGHT

Chakras are energetic bodies operating within the subtle energy system. Their main job is to transform physical energy into subtle energy and vice versa, so the "subtle us" can hum along in a state of well-being and happiness. When this occurs, our everyday lives are apt to be healthy and joyful too.

There are many definitions of *chakra*, but they all evolve from the Sanskrit meaning of the word: "wheel of light." Most authorities agree that chakras are located at the main branchings of the nervous system, where they serve as collection and transmission centers for both subtle (or metaphysical) energy and concrete (or biophysical) energy. As such, these centers tie together different parts of the body, the body with the cosmos, and all aspects of being—physical, emotional, mental, and spiritual—with one another. At the same time, each chakra performs its own unique function within the anatomical structure of the body's subtle system.

Chakras are envisioned as either circular or, when emerging from the body, as vortices that are conical in shape. According to various Sanskrit sources, a circle holds many meanings. For example, it describes a rotation of *shakti*, or feminine life energy, denotes *yantras* (mystical symbols) that direct reality, and references the different nerve centers in the body. These and other analyses of the word reduce to a simple definition of the word chakra:

*A chakra is a circular-shaped energy body that directs life energy for physical and spiritual well-being.*

Our forebears observed these subtle energy bodies, organs that convert fast-moving energy into slow-moving energy and vice versa, as connected through a network of energy channels called nadis. The chakras appear in hundreds of cultures across the globe, but the foremost authority on all things chakra is the Hindu tradition. Because of this, your coloring adventure will mainly involve learning about the seven main Hindu chakras—but keep your passport in hand. We'll also visit various other cultural ideas about the chakras and their subtle companions, the nadis.

As you'll discover, modern derivative chakra systems usually outline seven chakras, which ascend along the spine from the coccyx area to the top of the head. They are often affiliated with an aspect of consciousness or a major theme; a color; an element; a sound; a lotus (with differing numbers of petals); and interactions with the physical, emotional, mental, and spiritual aspects of being human. Each chakra is also frequently associated with a gland of the endocrine system and a nervous system nexus (plexus or ganglion).

Nearly every cultural chakra system considers the chakras a vital part of an enlightenment or spiritualization process. Chakras are fully awakened through the rise of *kundalini*, a life energy that rises from the lowest to the highest chakra. When the kundalini rises (through the nadis and up the spine), the chakras are cleansed and are able to more fully function physically, psychologically, and spiritually.

Most systems place the chakras at the same basic locations, as is done in this coloring book:

*First chakra:* Groin
*Second chakra:* Abdomen
*Third chakra:* Solar plexus
*Fourth chakra:* Heart
*Fifth chakra:* Throat
*Sixth chakra:* Forehead
*Seventh chakra:* In the top of the head

When you are coloring, know that many of the colors indicated have been chosen carefully. Most chakra systems denote chakras as vibratory bands of energy—or light—as well as sound. Each band is associated with a color, so whenever possible, use the colors selected for you.

Know also that each chakra is associated with dozens of different descriptors. You'll be introduced to several of these throughout this section, such as the following:

*Attribute:* The chakra's major characteristic

*Element:* Subtle energy creating material reality

*Granthi:* An energy knot composed of subtle energies that must be untied for the kundalini or life energy to rise

*Lotus petals:* A flower with strong symbolic meaning in Hindu philosophy; the number of petals reflects the movement of the chakra

*Seed syllable:* A *bija* or seed sound, the mystical mantra representing the chakra

*Yantra:* A geometric design or symbol facilitating meditation upon the chakra

Other terms will be explained as needed.

## CHAKRAS AND THE ENDOCRINE SYSTEM

Every chakra is linked with an endocrine gland and its corresponding system. Some chakra systems select different endocrine glands from others as the main organ; yet others emphasize supportive organs. Following is an outline of a few of the duties performed by the major glands. Described is the most widely accepted gland associated with a specific chakra, as well as alternative and supportive organs where applicable.

### First Chakra: Adrenals
The adrenal glands produce hormones vital to life and our reaction to stress.

### Second Chakra : Testes/ovaries
The gonads produce our sexual hormones and enable procreation.

### Third Chakra: Pancreas
The pancreas makes hormones and enzymes important for digestion and to regulate blood sugar. Some systems showcase the spleen, which manufactures red blood cells, as the major organ, and most include the liver, which cleanses the blood, as an important support organ. They also emphasize the kidneys, which balance cell salts and fluids, as support organs.

### Fourth Chakra: Heart
The heart provides the body with oxygen and nutrition; it's the center of the circulatory system. Some systems feature the thymus, which supports our immune system, as the main organ.

### Fifth Chakra: Thyroid
The thyroid manufactures hormones that regulate our metabolism and multiple organ functions. The parathyroid supports the thyroid.

### Sixth Chakra: Pituitary
The pituitary gland creates hormones for growth, metabolism, sexual function, and more.

### Seventh Chakra: Pineal
The pineal gland secretes hormones for mood and sleep, among other functions.

*See pages 72–73 for Chakras and the Endocrine System.*

## THE HINDU CHAKRA SYSTEM
The Hindu-based chakras are known by their Sanskrit names and are associated with specific colors. When you color in the titles of the pages that cover individual chakras, use their associated colors from the coloring instructions.

As the Hindu concepts of chakras developed over the centuries, each also become linked to a seed syllable, an element, and an attribute. Three chakras are also linked to granthis.

*See pages 74–75 for the Hindu Chakra System.*

### First chakra: Muladhara
Color: Red
Seed syllable: *Lam*

Element: Earth
Attribute: Patience
Granthi: *Brahma*

The Muladhara chakra, also called the first, base, or root chakra, is the first of the in-body chakras, lying at the base of the spine. From here arise the nadis, the subtle energy channels that carry life energy throughout the body. As such, the first chakra is considered the subtle energy center of the coccygeal nerve plexus but is also of vital importance in forming a physical and psychological foundation for our lives. This chakra contains the first of three granthis, or knots, that must be unbound to allow the kundalini to rise.

The depiction of the first chakra is crucial to understanding it. The lotus has four petals, which are all red. Within these is a yellow square, signifying the earth element. The yantra, or downward-pointed triangle within the square, reflects the feminine sexual organ. The symbol within these represents the seed syllable or mantra *lam*, which keeps our energy from moving below the first chakra in the body.

*See page 76 for the First Chakra.*

## Second chakra: Svadhisthana

Color: Orange
Seed syllable: *Vam*
Element: Water
Attribute: Purity

This chakra initiates the expansion of one's individuality. Its location at the sexual organs reflects the instinctual need to develop a specific personality but also to reach out to others. The watery element of this chakra encourages us to enjoy the rhythms and cycles of life and to express our psyche in all we do.

*See page 77 for the Second Chakra.*

## Third chakra: Manipura

Color: Yellow
Seed syllable: *Ram*
Element: Fire
Attribute: Radiance

The Manipura chakra presents itself as a brilliant, luminescent jewel. Elementally associated with fire, it is like a bright sun in the middle of the body. This center, which manages the digestive process and organs, also influences the nervous system and the immune process. Digestion is a reflection of the ability to digest and assimilate everything—including thoughts. Thus, this center determines the health of both our bodies and minds.

The third chakra is represented by a downward-pointing triangle, representing fire, within a circle. The ten petals of the lotus are blue—as blue as the center of a hot flame—or black. Within this chakra, we hear the sound *ram*.

*See page 78 for the Third Chakra.*

## Fourth chakra: Anahata

Color: Green
Seed syllable: *Yam*
Element: Air
Attribute: Contentment
Granthi: Vishnu

It is said that the enlightened can hear the sound of the universe within the Anahata chakra. Indeed, the heart is the center of the human body, the most vital human organ. The heart emanates thousands of times more electricity and magnetism than the brain does. Anahata's central organ, the heart, beats our existence with each pulse, revealing that, indeed, all of life is about sound and rhythm. The heart holds the second of the granthis, or locks, the knotted energies we must untangle if we are to free our divinity.

The heart is represented by two superimposed triangles within a circle, one pointing upward and the other pointing downward. These form a six-pointed star. The lotus has twelve petals, often seen as red, although the element, air, is gray in color. The emanating sound is *yam*.

*See page 79 for the Fourth Chakra.*

## Fifth chakra: Vishuddha

Color: Blue
Seed syllable: *Ham*
Element: Akasha (ether)
Attribute: Unity

Vishuddha is the center for communicating our truth to the world. It is about giving voice—or music or sound—to our inner heart and, in turn, hearing what the world has to reply. This is the last of the chakras that processes the gross or physical elements. Within its location, we prepare to ascend the ladder of consciousness, to shift into the chakras devoted to spirituality. It is time to ask what needs to be said to make this transcendence possible.

Symbolically, the fifth chakra looks like a downward-pointing triangle within a circle, which in turn encompasses a smaller circle. The lotus wears sixteen petals, which most systems present as violet blue. It is governed by ether, the most subtle of elements. The mantra *ham* energizes and harmonizes the throat.

*See page 80 for the Fifth Chakra.*

### Sixth chakra: Ajna
Color: Violet
Seed syllable: *Om*
Element: Supreme element
Attribute: Founding element
Granthi: Rudra

Solar and lunar energies meet and mix in the sixth chakra, combining the following principles: earthliness, liquidity, conscience, neutrality, austerity, violence, and spiritual devotion. The Ajna dissolves duality, allowing us to stop seeing "good" and "bad," to cease differentiating between "I" and "you," until we can accept the greater unity within the cosmos. Here we might draw upon our third eye, or inner sight, to peer through "reality" into the truth underneath. Herein lies the third granthi, or knot. Through its energy, we are invited to see everything as sacred.

Ajna is represented by a downward-pointing triangle within a circle. There are only two petals to its lotus. It is transparent and made of light, for its purpose is to help us see clearly. Its mantra is the divine *aum*, which connects the beginnings and endings of all things. This chakra is not associated with a specific element, although it is sometimes called the center of the supreme element—the light that generates all other elements. As such, it is usually considered to hold the seed syllable, *om*.

*See page 81 for the Sixth Chakra.*

### Seventh chakra: Sahasrara
Color: White
Seed syllable: None
Element: Beyond time and space
Attribute: Purity

Shiva and Shakti—the masculine and feminine—join within Sahasrara to create the transcendence of both. Within this chakra, the individual personality dissolves into the essence of the all. This is the chakra of one thousand petals. These petals represent the fifty letters of the Sanskrit alphabet along with their twenty permutations. The magnitude of these vibrations enhances the seventh chakra's role in governing and coordinating the other chakras.

This chakra is unique in many ways. All other chakras feature upward-pointing lotuses. In the Sahasrara, the lotuses point downward, symbolizing freedom from the mundane and divine rain from its petals. These petals are often shown with all the colors of the rainbow. The chakra is considered beyond most symbolic representations and elements, although the sound is frequently described as *visarga*, which is a breathing sound, or depicted with an *om*.

*See page 82 for the Seventh Chakra.*

## THE THREE MAIN NADIS

There are fourteen major nadis or subtle energy channels that connect the chakras and support the rising of the kundalini. Among these, there are three main nadis.

The *Sushumna* runs inside the vertebral column straight up from the base of the spine to the center of the brain. It feeds the major chakras, linking the first, or Muladhara, chakra to the seventh, or Sahasrara, chakra.

The *Ida* starts and ends on the left side of the body and is considered feminine and magnetic in nature. The *Pingala* starts and stops on the right side and is described as masculine and electrical. These two cross like a double helix and relate to the sympathetic nervous trunks on the sides of the spinal column. Together these two nadis interact to cleanse the physical body and to stimulate the rising of the kundalini through the Sushumna.

*See pages 84–85 for the Three Main Nadis.*

## THE TIBETAN SIX-CHAKRA SYSTEM

The Tibetan tradition describes six major chakras, each linked to one of six realms of existence or *lokas* and an element. Each chakra is also associated with a particular negative emotion and with a *buddha* whose positive qualities can purify or counteract the negativity of that loka. An individual performs yoga to tap into the positive qualities latent within these chakras, often using sound and visualization to activate the chakras' seed syllables, or mantras, and symbolic gestures as well as using practices to open dormant chakric powers.

In the system shown below, each chakra has a seed syllable representing one of the five elements (which are associated with specific colors); another representing the loka; and yet another representing the buddha whose qualities can purify the negativity of that loka.

In Tibetan culture, each element is represented by a color. The color assigned varies depending on the system, but one fairly common association follows:

> *Fire:* Red
> *Water:* Blue
> *Earth:* Yellow
> *Space:* White
> *Air:* Green

In the illustration on page 87, which is one of many examples representing Tibetan beliefs, each chakra is related to a different element, and the throat chakra is composed of all colors, or a rainbow. Your assignment is to color each chakra according to its representative element, as shown in the coloring instructions, page 86.

*See pages 86–87 for the Tibetan Six-Chakra System.*

## THE TSALAGI (CHEROKEE) SYSTEM

Many indigenous cultures carry knowledge of the subtle energies; among them are the traditional Tsalagi, the native term for the Cherokee people of North America.

According to the Tsalagi, we live in a field of mind that interconnects with the earth and the stars. To develop into our highest potential, we must send "fire" up the spine to animate the entire self. The spine is considered a ladder to heaven.

There are three fires that burn in the spine, each fulfilling a different purpose.

**Blue fire of will (blue)**
Clear intention to act

**Compassion fire (yellow)**
Understands and manifests purpose

**Fire of active intelligence (red)**
Acts in harmony

These three fires must penetrate the five doorways in the body where energy can become blocked. These doorways are reflective of the basic chakras:

**Solar plexus:** Here, one transforms feelings, such as anger, and negative thoughts in order to achieve higher action.

**Heart:** The heart holds the intellect. Around it are two electrical fields. One moves clockwise, the other counterclockwise. These generate purpose, the manifestation of dream in physical reality. To heal the heart is to become a balancing point between heaven and earth. This healing usually involves dealing with issues of compassion, grief, and fear.

**Throat:** Here is the power of the voice, the ability to say it and make it so. The key is to use this power wisely.

**Medulla:** The medulla rests at the base of the skull. It is a receptacle of past issues and problems, even those carried over from other lifetimes. This doorway invites the opportunity to live in the present.

**Crown:** Located in the fontanel, this gateway emits fluid once an aspirant has completed lessons, all of which center on nonattachment. This doorway formulates a full connection to the higher field of consciousness and the opportunity to fully embody the wisdom of the three burning fires.

## FOUR ADDITIONAL CENTERS

In addition to these five energy centers, there are four more: one in the "secret" region of the reproductive organs; one at the navel, which receives five subtle airs, five principles, five tones, and five rivers of color and sound that feed the five bodily organ systems, with each energy flowing one to the other from emptiness to sound (also called intention), from intention to wisdom, and from wisdom to love; one at the thymus; and one at the hands and feet, considered to be connected by a single energy that ascends one side of the body and descends the other.

*See pages 88–89 for the Tsalagi System.*

## OJOS DE LUZ: THE INCAN ENERGY SYSTEM

Although Incan-based energy systems differ, many propose a luminous energy field, called a *popo*, that surrounds our physical body. This luminous energy field is shaped like a bagel, mirroring the magnetic field of the earth. Energy flows out the top of the head to follow the luminous energy field, at which point it penetrates the earth for about twelve inches and reenters the body through our feet. The chakras are organs of this field.

Chakras are known in South America as *ojos de luz*, "eyes of light." The chakras extend threads of light, *huaskas*, that reach beyond the body, connecting the body to the natural world. These threads also reach backward and forward through time, from birth and personal history to our destination.

Like the Hindu, the Inca perceive seven chakras; however, they also describe two additional chakras. The eighth chakra is located above the physical body, but still within the luminous energy field. It is called the source of the sacred, *wiracocha*, our connection to the Creator. The ninth chakra, known as the *causay*, is outside the body and at one with all creation, the Creator's connection to each of us. The lower five chakras receive sustenance from the earth, and the upper four receive their nourishment from the sun.

All energy comes from five sources: plants and animals; water; air; sunlight; and biomagnetic energy, or causay.

*See pages 90–91 for the Incan Energy System.*

## INCAN BANDS OF POWER RITUAL

Incan shaman expert and renowned author Dr. Alberto Villoldo instructs students in the Bands of Power ritual in order to enable energetic protection. This process links six of the chakras to the five elements so that they may be nourished directly. It involves establishing five bands at various places in the body. Each band reflects the color of the element.

*See pages 92–93 for the Incan Bands of Power Ritual.*

## THE TWELVE-CHAKRA SYSTEM AND ENERGY EGG

One contemporary chakra system is the Twelve-Chakra System, which is based on the classical Hindu chakra system but includes an additional five chakras that are outside of the physical body. The additional chakras are found above the head, below the feet, and around the body. As with the traditional systems that describe fewer chakras, each chakra within the twelve-chakra universe governs specific physical functions. Additionally, each chakra performs a particular overall mission and is linked to an auric field that surrounds the body.

The final boundary of the auric field is an "energy egg," a three-layered electromagnetic body that surrounds and penetrates the twelve chakras and auric bands.

### First chakra
Genital organs and adrenals; coccygeal vertebrae; affects some kidney, bladder, and excretory functions; skin
*Mission:* Security and survival

### Second chakra
Affects part of adrenal system; intestines; parts of kidney function; some aspects of reproductive system; sacral vertebrae and the neurotransmitters determining emotional responses to stimuli
*Mission:* Feelings and creativity

### Third chakra
Pancreatic system; all digestive organs in stomach area, including liver, spleen, gallbladder, stomach, pancreas, and parts of kidney system; lumbar vertebrae
*Mission:* Mentality and structure

### Fourth chakra
Heart and lungs; circulatory and oxygenation systems; breasts; lumbar and thoracic vertebrae
*Mission:* Relationships and healing

### Fifth chakra
Thyroid gland; larynx; mouth and auditory systems; lymph system; thoracic vertebrae
*Mission:* Communication and guidance

### Sixth chakra
Pituitary gland; parts of hypothalamus; visual and olfactory systems; memory storage; some problems with ears and sinus; left eye
*Mission:* Vision and strategy

### Seventh chakra
Pineal gland; parts of hypothalamus; higher learning and cognitive brain systems; parts of immune system; right eye
*Mission:* Purpose and spirituality

### Eighth chakra
Thymus (immune system); memory retrieval functions; aspects of central nervous system; thalamus
*Mission:* Karma and universal linkages

### Ninth chakra
Diaphragm; pineal gland; corpus callosum and other higher learning centers including the cortex and neocortex
*Mission:* Soul programs and plans

### Tenth chakra
Feet, legs, and bones
*Mission:* Legacies and nature

### Eleventh chakra
Parts of skin, muscles, and connective tissue
*Mission:* Forces and energy conversion

### Twelfth chakra
Secondary chakric sites that include the knees, elbows, palms, and organs; layer that connects to energy egg
*Mission:* Ending human self; access to energy egg

### Energy Egg Layers

**Inside layer**
Supports physical manifestation

**Middle layer**
Opens to possibilities

**Outer layer**
Accesses spiritual realms

*See pages 94–95 for the Twelve-Chakra System.*

# CHAKRAS AND THE ENDOCRINE SYSTEM

Color in all the chakra areas and organs related to each chakra. Some of the chakras will have supportive or secondary organs in addition to the main organ.

## FIRST CHAKRA

ADRENALS red

## SECOND CHAKRA

TESTES/OVARIES orange

## THIRD CHAKRA

PANCREAS yellow

ALTERNATIVE ORGAN
SPLEEN yellow

SUPPORT ORGAN
LIVER yellow

## FOURTH CHAKRA

HEART green

ALTERNATIVE ORGAN
THYMUS green

## FIFTH CHAKRA

THYROID medium blue

SECONDARY ORGAN
PARATHYROID medium blue

## SIXTH CHAKRA

PITUITARY violet

## SEVENTH CHAKRA

PINEAL white

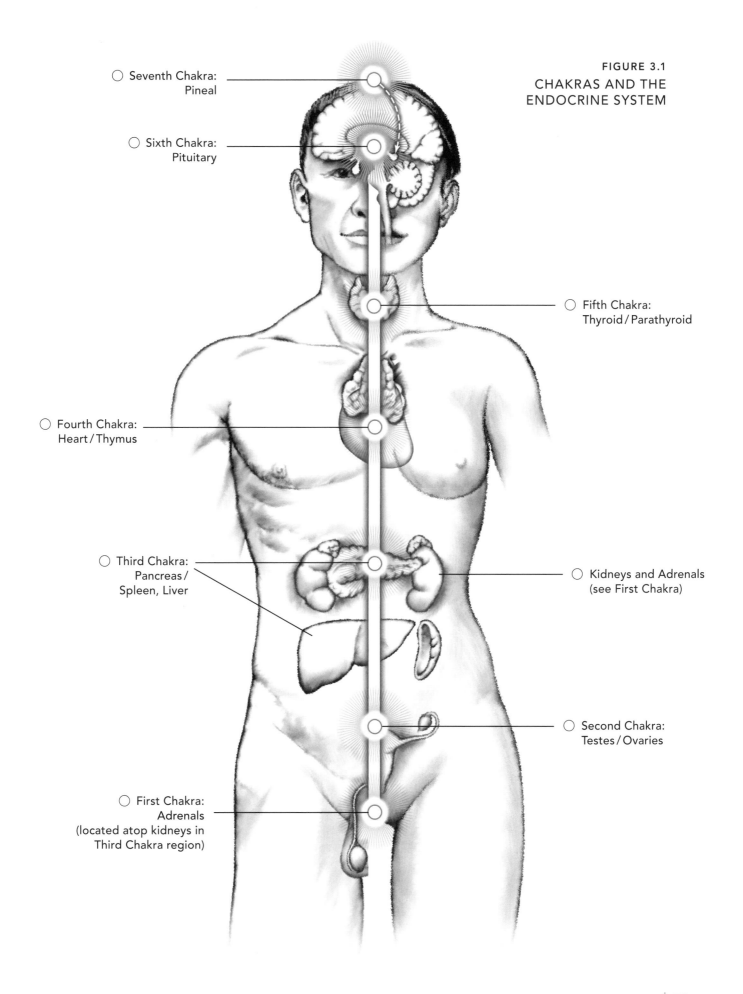

FIGURE 3.1
CHAKRAS AND THE
ENDOCRINE SYSTEM

○ Seventh Chakra:
Pineal

○ Sixth Chakra:
Pituitary

○ Fifth Chakra:
Thyroid / Parathyroid

○ Fourth Chakra:
Heart / Thymus

○ Third Chakra:
Pancreas /
Spleen, Liver

○ Kidneys and Adrenals
(see First Chakra)

○ Second Chakra:
Testes / Ovaries

○ First Chakra:
Adrenals
(located atop kidneys in
Third Chakra region)

# HINDU CHAKRA SYSTEM

Color the body-based chakra and its name with the colors below.

| | | |
|---|---|---|
| MULADHARA | FIRST CHAKRA | red |
| SVADHISTHANA | SECOND CHAKRA | orange |
| MANIPURA | THIRD CHAKRA | yellow |
| ANAHATA | FOURTH CHAKRA | green |
| VISHUDDHA | FIFTH CHAKRA | blue |
| AJNA | SIXTH CHAKRA | violet |
| SAHASRARA | SEVENTH CHAKRA | white |

FIGURE 3.2
THE HINDU CHAKRA SYSTEM

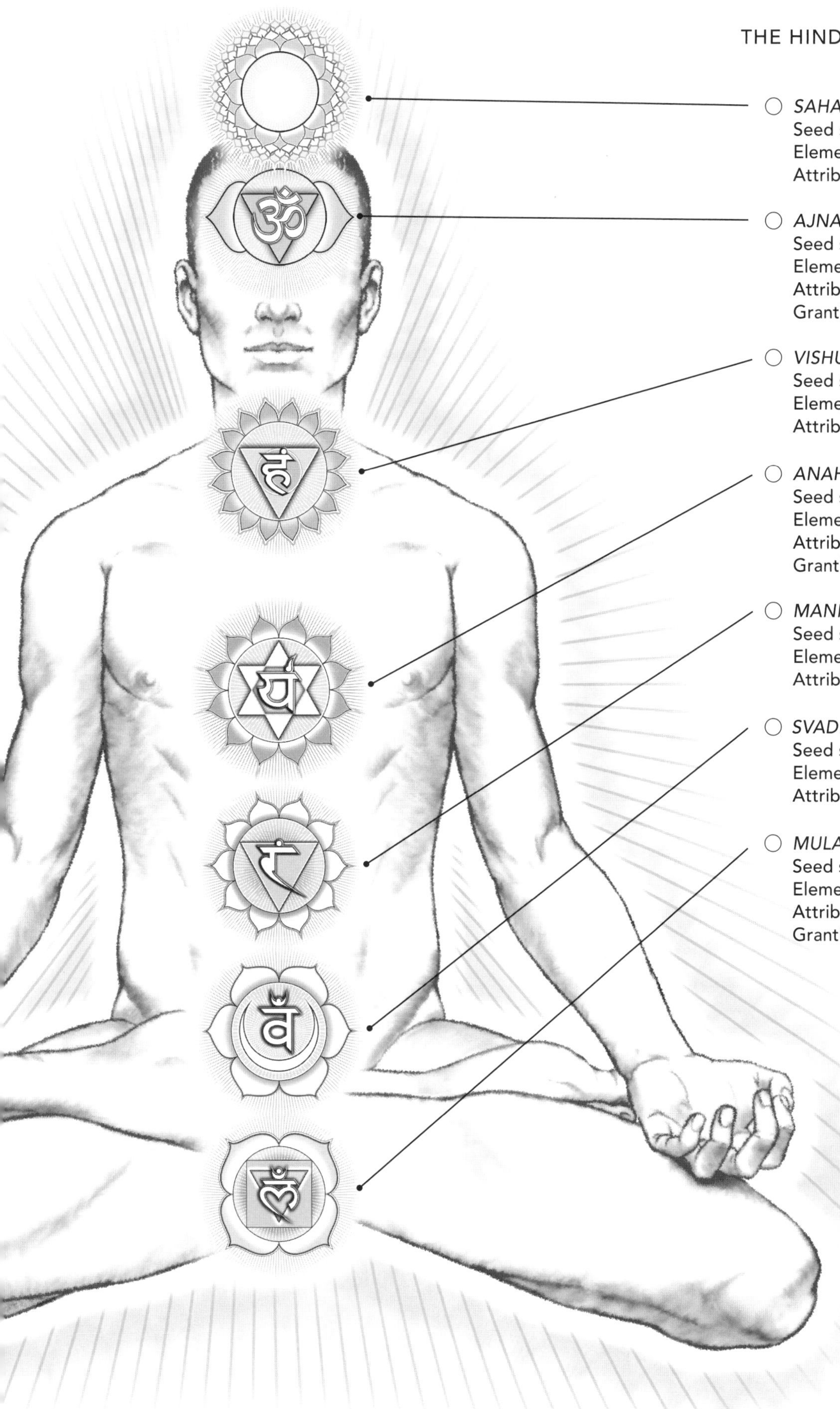

○ *SAHASRARA*
Seed syllable: None
Element: Beyond time and space
Attribute: Purity

○ *AJNA*
Seed syllable: *Om*
Element: Supreme element
Attribute: Founding element
Granthi: Rudra

○ *VISHUDDHA*
Seed syllable: *Ham*
Element: Akasha (ether)
Attribute: Unity

○ *ANAHATA*
Seed syllable: *Yam*
Element: Air
Attribute: Contentment
Granthi: Vishnu

○ *MANIPURA*
Seed syllable: *Ram*
Element: Fire
Attribute: Radiance

○ *SVADHISTHANA*
Seed syllable: *Vam*
Element: Water
Attribute: Purity

○ *MULADHARA*
Seed syllable: *Lam*
Element: Earth
Attribute: Patience
Granthi: Brahma

# FIRST CHAKRA: MULADHARA

Color: Red  •  Seed syllable: *Lam*  •  Element: Earth  •  Attribute: Patience  •  Granthi: Brahma

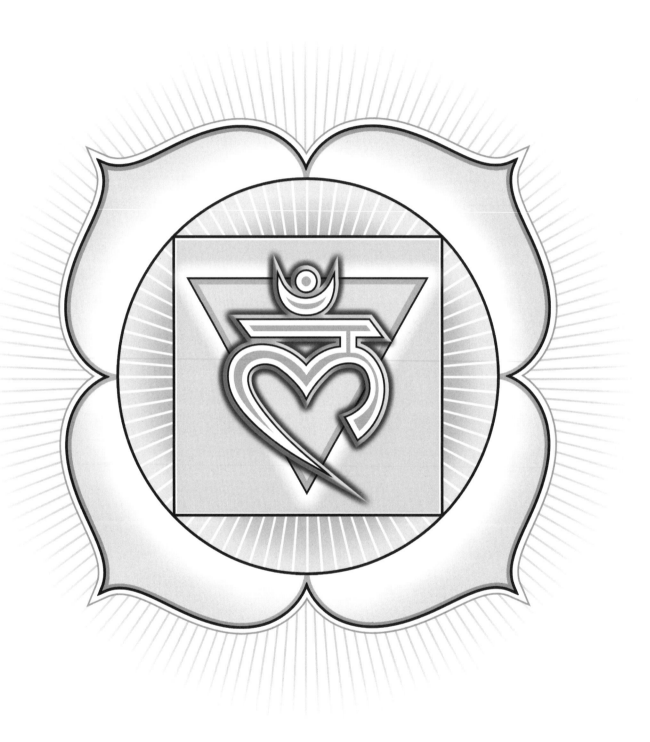

**FIGURE 3.3**

Coloring Instructions: Use red for the title of the page. Outline the square and triangle with yellow. Also use gold to outline and fill in the mantra: the symbol within the square. Use red with a tint of yellow (to make vermilion) to color in the four lotus petals that surround the square. Fill in the remainder of chakra and the label with red.

# SECOND CHAKRA: SVADHISTHANA

Color: Orange • Seed syllable: *Vam* • Element: Water • Attribute: Purity

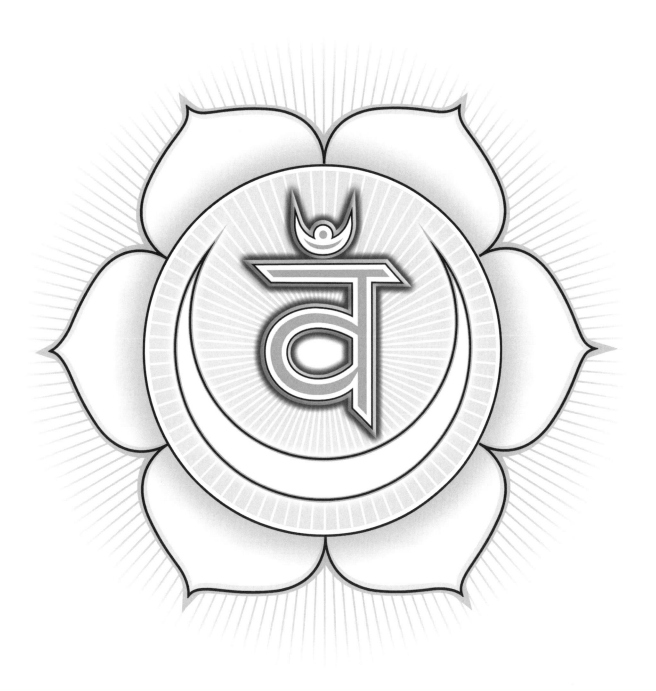

**FIGURE 3.4**

Coloring Instructions: Use orange for the title of the page. Use white for the circle, silver for the moon, gold for the mantra, red and orange for the petals, and orange for the rest of the chakra.

# THIRD CHAKRA: MANIPURA

Color: Yellow • Seed syllable: *Ram* • Element: Fire • Attribute: Radiance

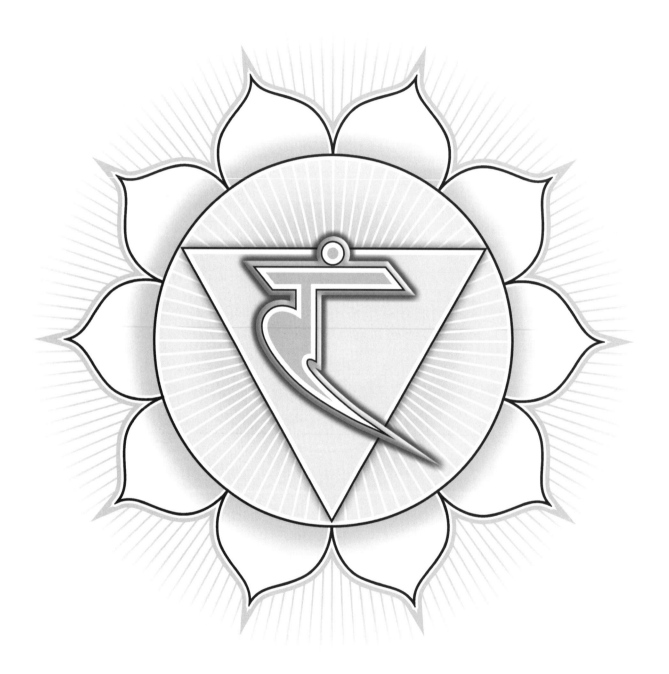

**FIGURE 3.5**

Coloring Instructions: Use yellow for the title of the page. Use red for the triangle, yellow for the circle, gold for the mantra, medium blue or black for the petals, and yellow for the rest of the chakra.

# FOURTH CHAKRA: ANAHATA

Color: Green • Seed syllable: *Yam* • Element: Air • Attribute: Contentment • Granthi: Vishnu

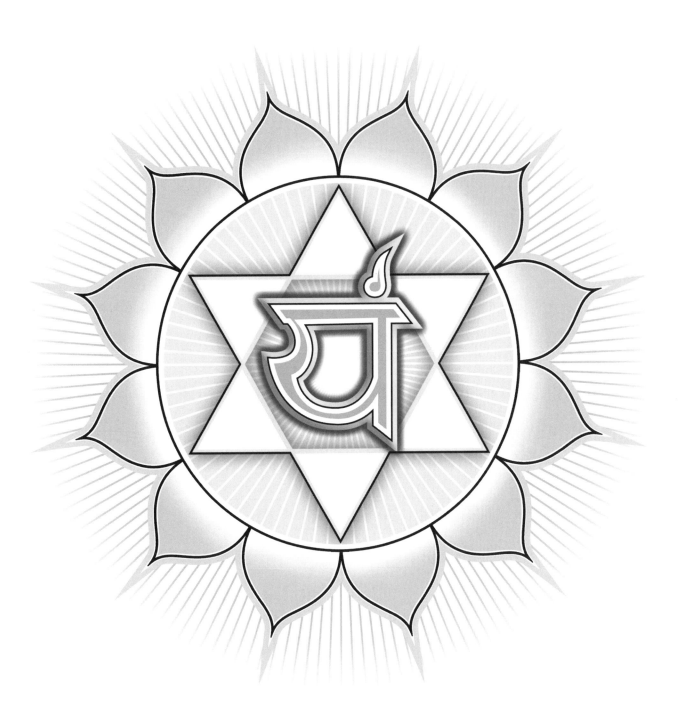

**FIGURE 3.6**

Coloring Instructions: Use green for the title of the page. Use gray for the star, gold for the mantra, red and black for the petals, and green for the rest of the chakra.

# FIFTH CHAKRA: VISHUDDHA

Color: Blue • Seed syllable: *Ham* • Element: Akasha (Ether) • Attribute: Unity

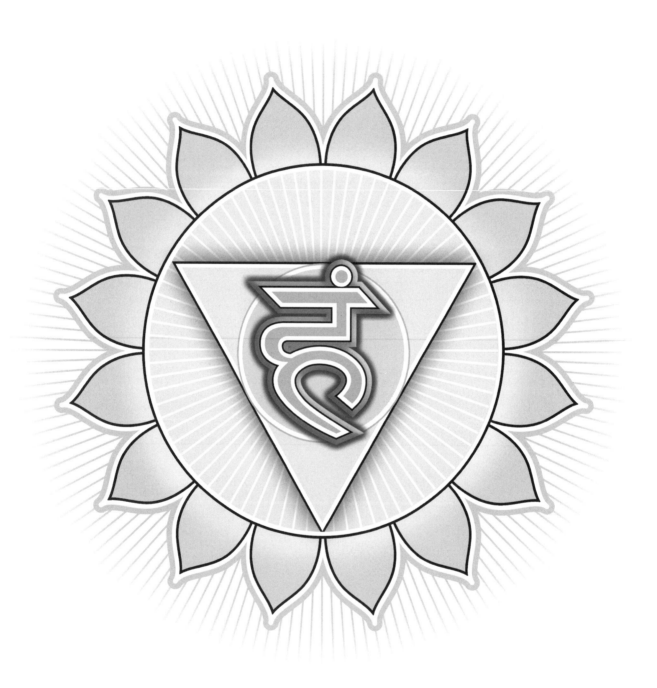

**FIGURE 3.7**

Coloring Instructions: Use medium blue for the title of the page. Use light blue for the triangle, silver for the outer circle, white for the inner circle, gold for the mantra, gray for the petals, and medium blue for the rest of the chakra.

# SIXTH CHAKRA: AJNA

Color: Violet   •   Seed syllable: *Om*   •   Element: Supreme element   •   Attribute: Founding element   •   Granthi: Rudra

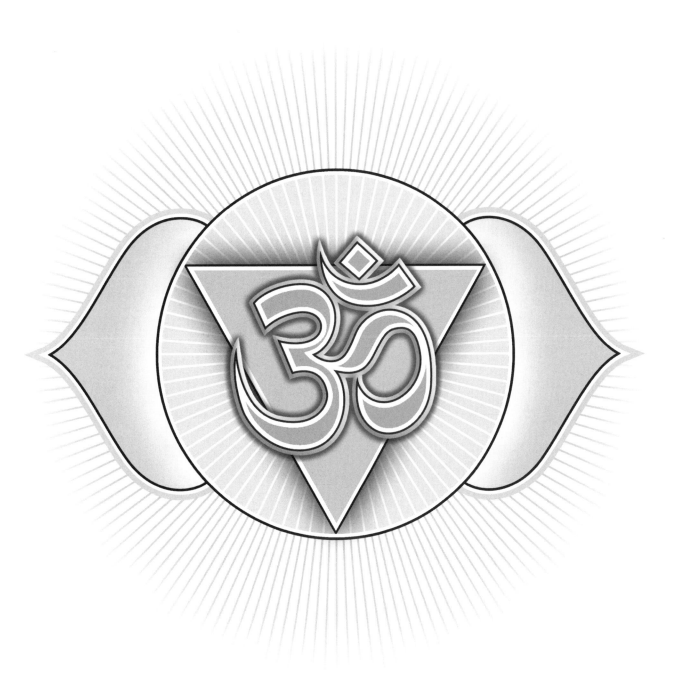

**FIGURE 3.8**

Coloring Instructions: Use violet for the title of the page. Use white for the triangle, white for the circle, gold for the mantra, white for the petals, and violet for the rest of the chakra.

# SEVENTH CHAKRA: SAHASRARA

Color: white  •  Seed syllable: None  •  Element: Beyond time and space  •  Attribute: Purity

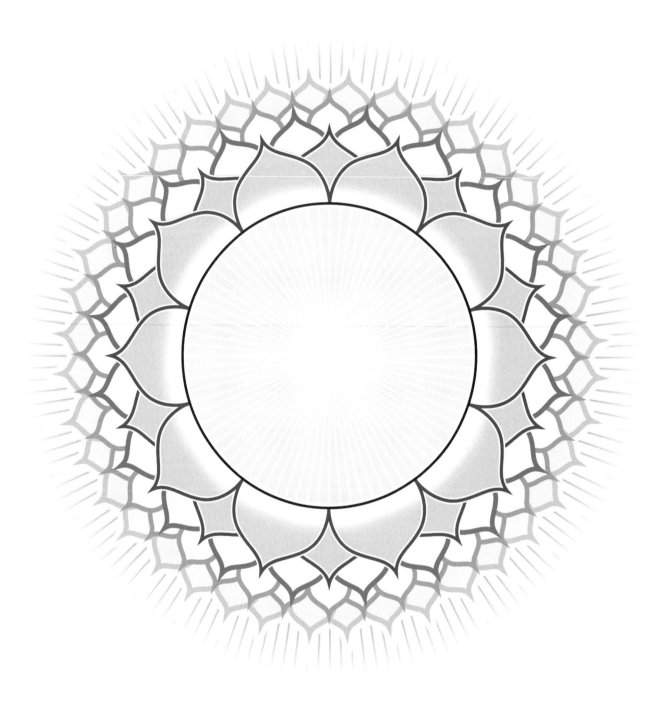

**FIGURE 3.9**

Coloring Instructions: Use white for the title of the page. Use red, orange, yellow, green, medium blue, violet, and white in rainbow sequence for the petals; and white for the rest of the chakra.

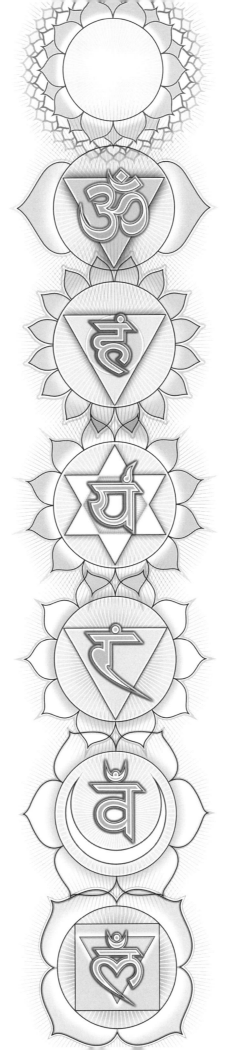

*A chakra is a circular-shaped energy body that directs life energy for physical and spiritual well-being.*

# THREE MAIN NADIS

Color the body-based chakra and its name with the colors below. Color the nadis with the suggested colors. Use yellow for the rays.

NADIS

IDA  silver

PINGALA  gold

SUSHUMNA  pink

CHAKRAS

FIRST CHAKRA  red

SECOND CHAKRA  orange

THIRD CHAKRA  yellow

FOURTH CHAKRA  green

FIFTH CHAKRA  medium blue

SIXTH CHAKRA  violet

SEVENTH CHAKRA  white

OTHER

RISING KUNDALINI  red

**FIGURE 3.10**
THE THREE MAIN NADIS

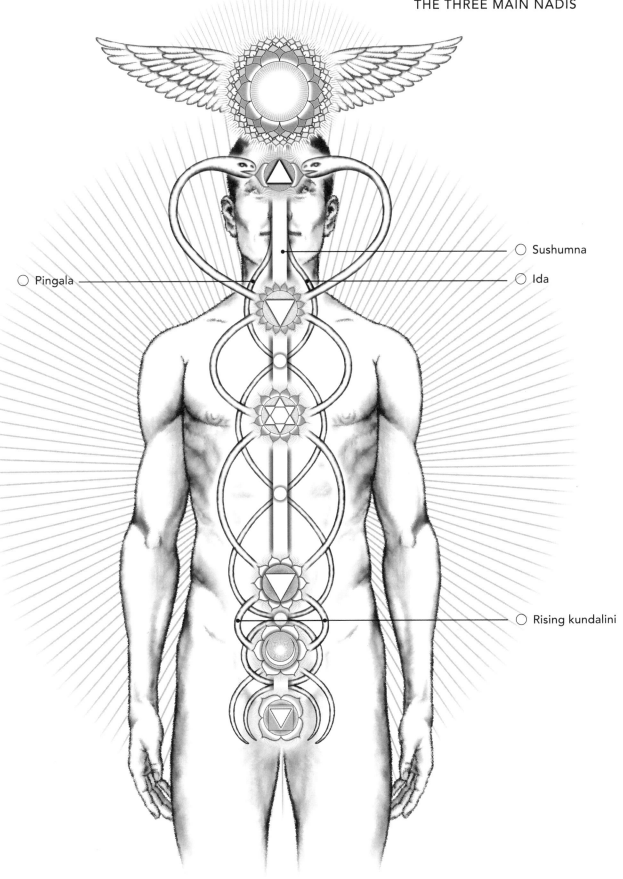

Sushumna

Ida

Pingala

Rising kundalini

# TIBETAN SIX-CHAKRA SYSTEM

In this illustration, which is one of many examples representing Tibetan beliefs, each chakra is related to a different element, and the throat chakra is composed of all colors, or a rainbow. Your assignment is to color each chakra according to its representative element, as follows. Use gold for the surrounding energy field.

## THROAT CHAKRA

Primordial syllable: *A*
Antidote: Peace

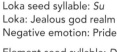

Loka seed syllable: *Su*
Loka: Jealous god realm
Negative emotion: Pride

Element seed syllable: *Drum*
Element: All five elements
Color: All five colors

## CROWN CHAKRA

Primordial syllable: *A*
Antidote: Compassion and joyful effort

Loka seed syllable: *A*
Loka: God realm
Negative emotion: Self-centeredness/lethargic pleasure

Element seed syllable: *Ham*
Element: Space
Color: White

## NAVEL CHAKRA

Primordial syllable: *A*
Antidote: Wisdom

Loka seed syllable: *Tri*
Loka: Animal realm
Negative emotion: Ignorance

Element seed syllable: *Mam*
Element: Water
Color: Medium blue

## HEART CHAKRA

Primordial syllable: *A*
Antidote: Openness

Loka seed syllable: *Ni*
Loka: Human realm
Negative emotion: Jealousy

Element seed syllable: *Kham*
Element: Earth
Color: Yellow

## LEFT FOOT CHAKRA

Primordial syllable: *A*
Antidote: Love

Loka seed syllable: *Du*
Loka: Hell realm
Negative emotion: Hatred

Element seed syllable: *Yam*
Element: Air
Color: Green

## RIGHT FOOT CHAKRA

Primordial syllable: *A*
Antidote: Love

Loka seed syllable: *Du*
Loka: Hell realm
Negative emotion: Hatred

Element seed syllable: *Yam*
Element: Air
Color: Green

## SECRET CHAKRA

Primordial syllable: *A*
Antidote: Generosity

Loka seed syllable: *Tri*
Loka: Hungry ghost realm
Negative emotion: Greed

Element seed syllable: *Ram*
Element: Fire
Color: Red

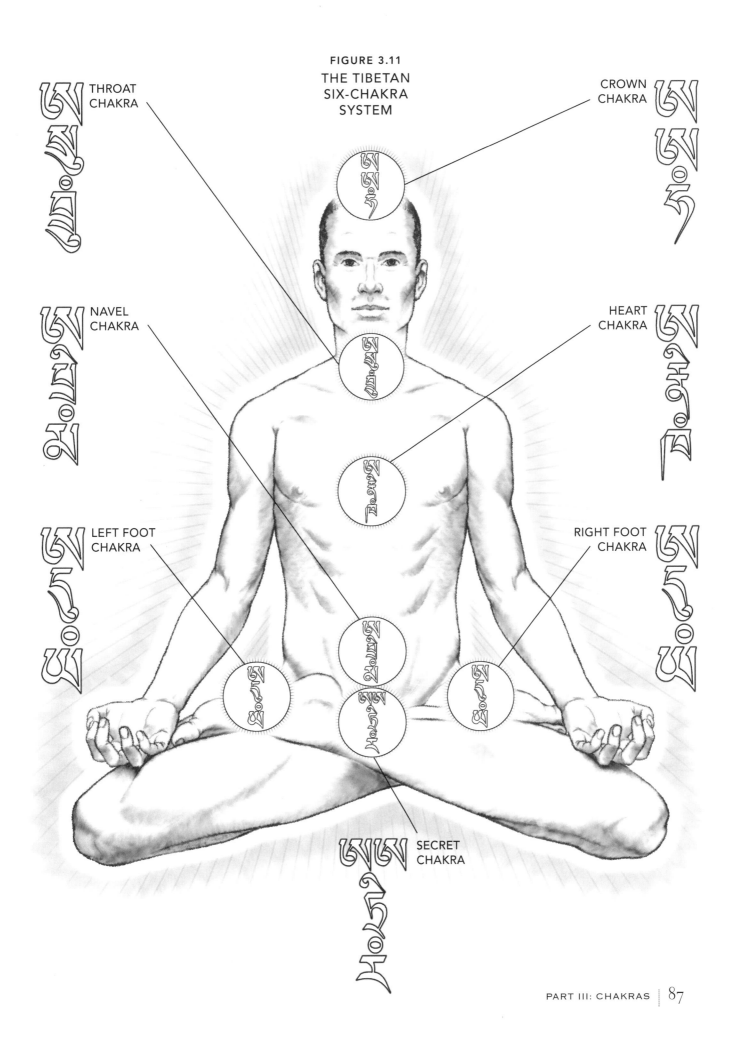

FIGURE 3.11
THE TIBETAN
SIX-CHAKRA
SYSTEM

CROWN
CHAKRA

THROAT
CHAKRA

HEART
CHAKRA

NAVEL
CHAKRA

LEFT FOOT
CHAKRA

RIGHT FOOT
CHAKRA

SECRET
CHAKRA

# THE TSALAGI (CHEROKEE) SYSTEM

The colors and symbols selected reflect the meaning of the ancient Tsalagi ideas of the sacred energy centers or chakras. However, if you feel drawn to do so, feel free to select a different color from the ones provided below.

## CROWN  Wisdom

Use yellow for the lines of the triangle and gold for the center of the triangle.

## THYMUS  Awakening through understanding

Use red, orange, yellow, green, medium blue, violet, and white in a rainbow spectrum for the torus.

## MEDULLA  Time

Use violet for the infinity sign.

## THROAT  Manifesting

Use violet for the star and deep blue or indigo for the half circle/crescent.

## HEART  Intellect

Use orange for the pyramids and gold for the wavy lines.

## SOLAR PLEXUS  Transformation

Use brown for the star; violet for the lines of the square; and a pastel color of your choice for the inside of the square.

## NAVEL  Five rivers and five airs

Use green for the circle and a pastel color of your choice for the streams of energy emanating from it.

## SECRET  Three fires

Use silver for the triangle inside of the area; and red, yellow, and medium blue for each of the three corners of the triangle.

## HANDS AND FEET  Surrounding energy

Use gold for the hands and feet and surrounding energy.

FIGURE 3.12
THE TSALAGI (CHEROKEE)
SYSTEM

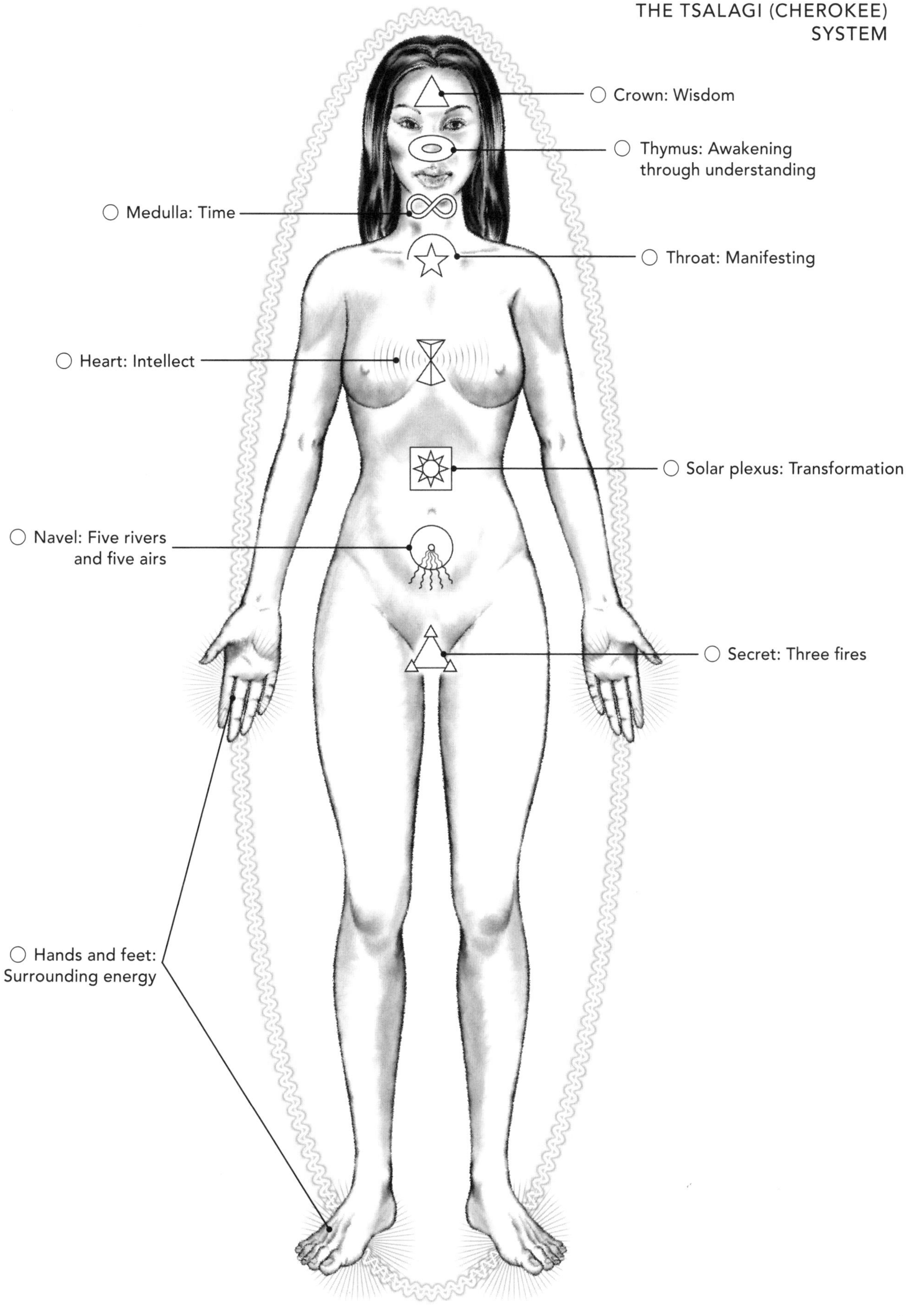

Crown: Wisdom

Thymus: Awakening
through understanding

Medulla: Time

Throat: Manifesting

Heart: Intellect

Solar plexus: Transformation

Navel: Five rivers
and five airs

Secret: Three fires

Hands and feet:
Surrounding energy

# OJOS DE LUZ: THE INCAN ENERGY SYSTEM

Color the chakra and its name with the colors below. Then color the huascas and additional terms as indicated.

HUASCAS  silver

PLANTS  green

LAND  brown

PEOPLE  pink

ANIMALS  pastel color of your choice

EARTH  light blue

LUMINOUS FIELD  gold

## CHAKRAS

FIRST CHAKRA  red

SECOND CHAKRA  orange

THIRD CHAKRA  yellow

FOURTH CHAKRA  green

FIFTH CHAKRA  medium blue

SIXTH CHAKRA  deep blue or indigo

SEVENTH CHAKRA  violet

EIGHTH CHAKRA  gold

NINTH CHAKRA  white

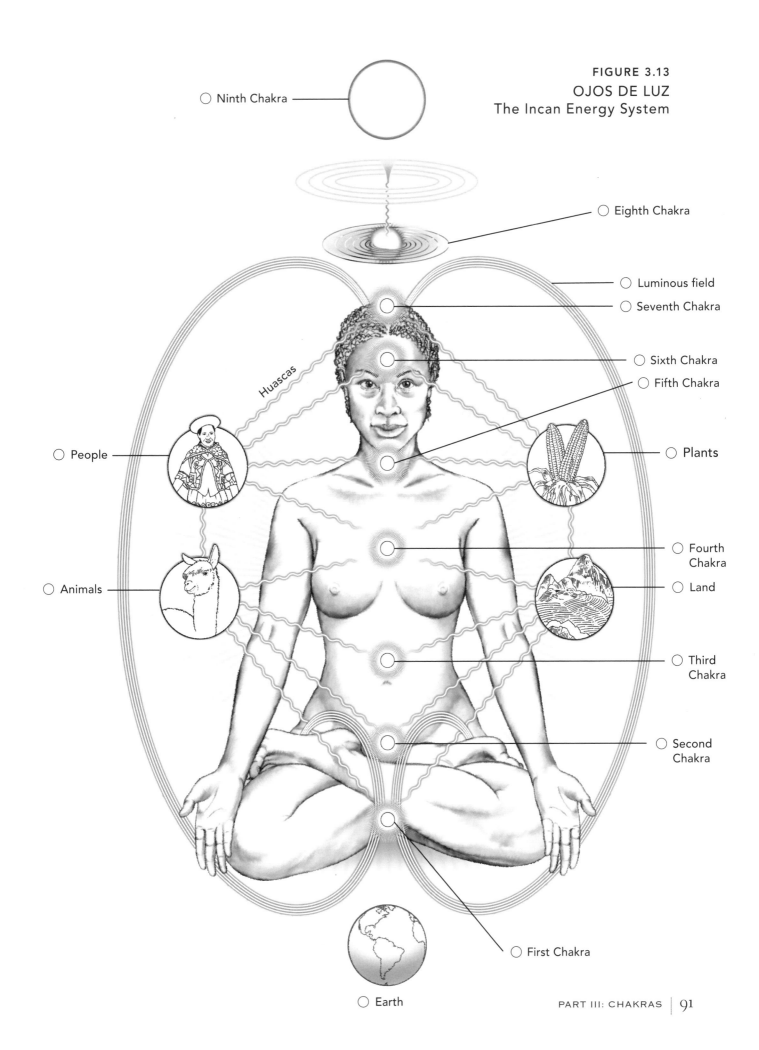

FIGURE 3.13

OJOS DE LUZ
The Incan Energy System

Ninth Chakra

Eighth Chakra

Luminous field
Seventh Chakra

Sixth Chakra
Fifth Chakra

Huascas

People

Plants

Fourth Chakra

Animals

Land

Third Chakra

Second Chakra

First Chakra

Earth

# INCAN BANDS OF POWER RITUAL

Color the body-based chakra band and its name with the colors below.

BANDS OF POWER

FIRST CHAKRA

EARTH ELEMENT black

SECOND & THIRD CHAKRA

WATER ELEMENT red

FOURTH CHAKRA

FIRE ELEMENT gold

FIFTH CHAKRA

WIND ELEMENT silver

SIXTH CHAKRA

UNIVERSE white

**FIGURE 3.14**
**INCAN BANDS OF
POWER RITUAL**

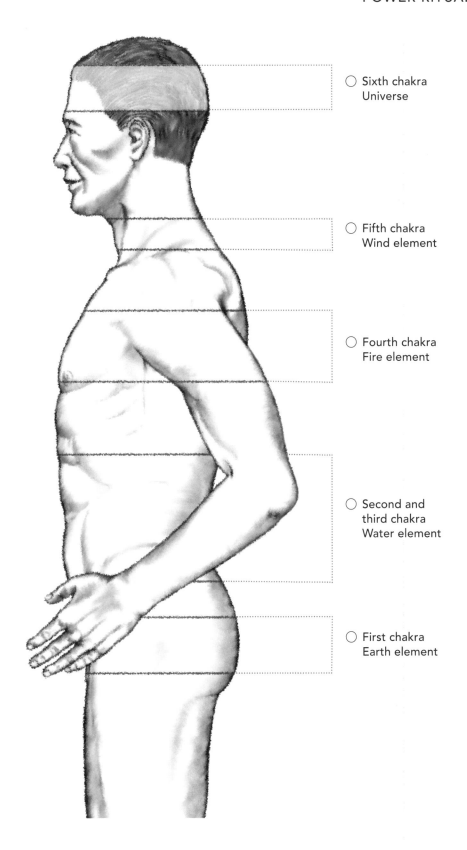

○ Sixth chakra
Universe

○ Fifth chakra
Wind element

○ Fourth chakra
Fire element

○ Second and
third chakra
Water element

○ First chakra
Earth element

# THE TWELVE-CHAKRA SYSTEM AND ENERGY EGG

Coloring Instructions: Use the recommended colors below to fill in the outlined words on this page, the circle next to the label on the facing page, and the associated part of the image. For the Twelfth Chakra, color the wavy lines that connect to the Energy Egg.

**CHAKRAS**

FIRST CHAKRA red

SECOND CHAKRA orange

THIRD CHAKRA yellow

FOURTH CHAKRA green

FIFTH CHAKRA medium blue

SIXTH CHAKRA violet

SEVENTH CHAKRA white

EIGHTH CHAKRA black

NINTH CHAKRA gold

TENTH CHAKRA brown

ELEVENTH CHAKRA pink

TWELFTH CHAKRA silver

**ENERGY EGG LAYERS**

INSIDE LAYER light blue

MIDDLE LAYER deep blue or indigo

OUTER LAYER gray

**FIGURE 3.15**
THE TWELVE-CHAKRA SYSTEM
AND ENERGY EGG

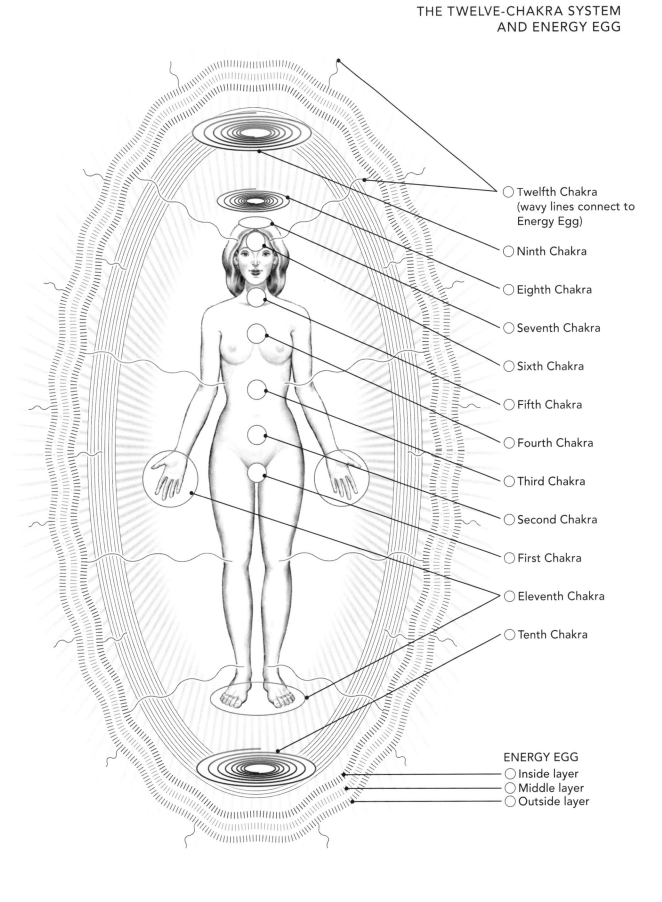

○ Twelfth Chakra
(wavy lines connect to
Energy Egg)

○ Ninth Chakra

○ Eighth Chakra

○ Seventh Chakra

○ Sixth Chakra

○ Fifth Chakra

○ Fourth Chakra

○ Third Chakra

○ Second Chakra

○ First Chakra

○ Eleventh Chakra

○ Tenth Chakra

ENERGY EGG
○ Inside layer
○ Middle layer
○ Outside layer

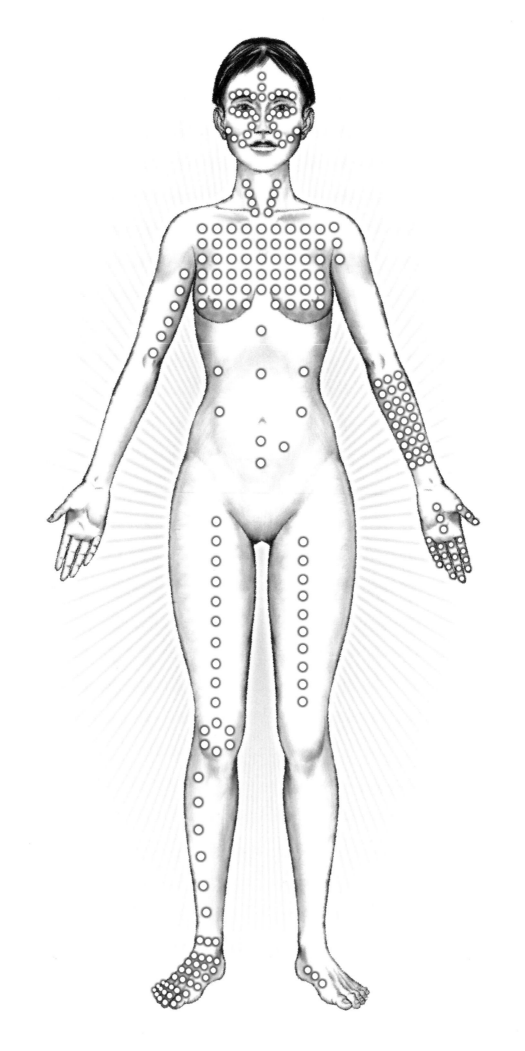

# PART IV
## SUBTLE ENERGY POINTS

There are many healing systems that promote balance by influencing the body's subtle energy points. We first introduced these in Part II as acupoints. In this section, we will explore three major healing systems that use these points.

On the first leg of the survey, we examine Shiatsu, a hands-on therapy from Japan that involves the manipulation of subtle energy points called *tsubo* points. We then visit Thailand to investigate the Thai energy system, which involves working on pressure points as well as chakras and energy channels. Then we round the corner to complete our survey of Traditional Chinese Medicine (TCM), which we also first mentioned in Part II.

In TCM, the acupoints are located on the meridians. At these points, the chi rises to the surface of the body. In Part II, you colored some of the most significant points that appear on individual meridians. But there are other types of subtle energy points, which might be labeled pressure points, reflex points, or zones, that are found on the feet, hands, head, and ears. In fact, specific points in these bodily areas correspond to bodily organs, systems of organs, and other parts of the body. In a process called reflexology, a practitioner can apply pressure to these subtle points and work the entire body or focus on a particular organ or system. In this section, you'll be introduced to the basic reflexology charts and points.

### BASIC SHIATSU POINTS

Shiatsu is a hands-on therapy that uses the palms, thumbs, and fingers to deliver healing through pressure,

a process effectively described by its name: *shi* means "finger," and *atsu* means "pressure." Shiatsu focuses on particular sections of the body to correct bodily imbalances and promote health. It is also considered a viable way to heal specific illnesses.

Shiatsu is similar to Traditional Chinese Medicine in that it focuses on specific bodily locations. Unlike TCM, however, the most strategic of these points are based at anatomically functional sites rather than energetically based areas. They are called tsubo points, meaning "vital point" or "important place." Many of these points, however, do interface with the traditional meridian points. Another difference between the two systems is that in Shiatsu, these points are unnamed.

Shiatsu was invented by a young Japanese boy, Tokujiro Namikoshi, in 1912. When he was seven years old, he cured his mother of rheumatism using only his thumbs, fingers, palms, and the application of pressure. As he matured, he discovered the 660 basic points, which he linked to bodily parts and functions through his studies in anatomy and physiology.

There are many other versions of Shiatsu, some of which include principles and practices from TCM, Zen Buddhism, and other forms of Buddhism. The diagrams you will color showcase the main tsubo points.

*See page 100–102 for the basic Shiatsu Points.*

### KEIKETSU SHIATSU POINTS

A Shiatsu session focuses mainly on the basic points but can also involve the *keiketsu* points, considered secondary points. The keiketsu points are in the same places as the acupoints of the meridians. Because of this, they are labeled with Chinese terms.

A practitioner works with these points to address specific symptoms and problems. Because of this, they are considered pathological reflex points. For instance, stimulating one of these points can potentially relieve a specific bodily pain or organic disorder. If pressed inappropriately, the body can also be harmed, at least temporarily. While these points are secondary, they are also powerful.

*See page 103 for the Keiketsu Shiatsu Points.*

## THAI ENERGY SYSTEM

Thai massage is an ancient healing process based on energy lines as well as the chakras. Thai massage channels differ somewhat in locality from those employed by Shiatsu and practitioners of Chinese medicine, although they are all described as working energetically and physically in much the same ways.

Most Thai massage scholars state that there are ten main lines, called *sen*, but they do not agree on their locations. There are three major types of lines: main, extension, and branch. While noting how these compare to the Hindu nadis and the meridians, follow the coloring instructions also provided.

> **Sen Sumana:**
> Identical to the Hindu Sushumna nadi and a combination of the Ren Mai and Du Mai channels of the Chinese tradition
>
> **Sen Ittha and Sen Pingkhala:**
> Related to the Hindu Ida and Pingala nadis and the Bladder meridian of the Chinese system
>
> **Sen Sahatsarangsi and Sen Thawari:**
> Combine to form the Chinese Stomach meridian

The sen are comparable to rivers of energy, and the chakras to whirlpools in the rivers. The seven major chakras are positioned along the centerline, or Sen Sumana, and several minor chakras are peppered around the body. Thai massage uses pressure points, which are not formally labeled but relate to the areas they affect and the disorders they address.

The illustrations on pages 107 and 109 show the ten main sen lines used in Thai massage according to the system developed by the authors of *The Art of Traditional Thai Massage: Energy Line Charts*. It also depicts the main lines and the chakras and briefly lists a few of the ailments pertaining to each sen line.

*See pages 104–109 for the Thai Energy System.*

## REFLEXOLOGY

Reflexology involves applying pressure to reflex points for stress relief, healing, and transformation. While some of these are also acupoints, there are many other subtle energy points as well, related to organs, glands, nerves and nerve ganglions (the latter are associated with the chakras in some systems), muscle groups, and bodily parts and systems. The four areas of the body that contain these representative points are the feet, hands, head, and ears.

Reflexology is believed to reduce pain and stress, alleviate psychological disturbances, and impact major illnesses. The goal is to bring the entire body into balance. As you color in the points, check to see if you are drawn to applying light pressure to any of them on your own body. After identifying the point or zone you want to engage, find it on yourself and apply gentle but firm pressure, but not to the level of feeling pain. For up to a few minutes, work this area with a thumb or your fingers. You can either apply steady pressure, or you can pulse the pressure—press and release, press and release.

Note that in this section, the colors are inconsistently assigned, although they will match the chakra area colors when applicable. Charts that are partnered will also share similar colors for the like body areas. For instance, the colors describing the bodily areas for the following section, "Foot Reflexology: Top of the Foot," are the same as those used for "Foot Reflexology: Sole of the Foot." In general, there are no standard metaphysical colors for many of the bodily areas.

Head reflexology works with zones or areas that affect certain body points as well as smaller, specific points. Also, certain zones are described by their location, such as "eye zone" and "ear zone."

*See pages 110–125 for Reflexology.*

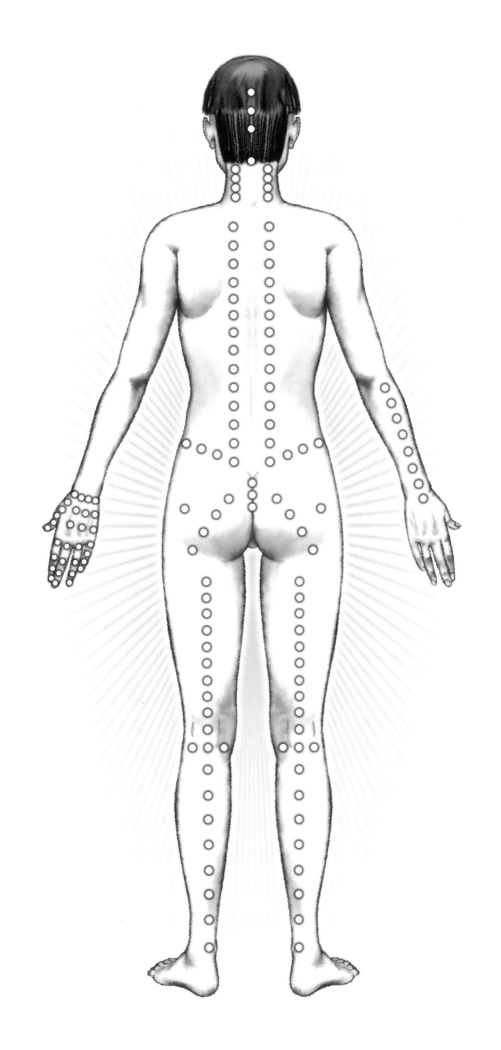

# BASIC SHIATSU POINTS: SIDE

Coloring Instructions: Use orange inside each point and yellow for the rims. Then do the exercise.

## EXERCISE

Want to work on a Shiatsu point with color? Shiatsu practitioners usually diagnose and treat with their thumbs, also applying palm- and hand-based pressures. They use techniques including shaking, rotating, patting, lifting, pinching, brushing, and more for healing.

As we explored in the section "The Meanings of Colors" in the introductory material in this book, every color has meaning. After coloring all the points, touch various points with your thumb until you discover a sensitive one. Imagine this point as red, the color of inflammation. Return to the illustration and draw a red circle around the related point. Get creative. Make it smooth, jagged, erratic, bold, or light, describing the pain with your depiction. Now imagine yourself sending blue or green energy into the inflamed point, keeping your thumb on the area. Blue is a cooling color and green is a healing hue. Grab a blue or green color—or both—and use them in relation to the red circle you colored around the point on the illustration. You can color over the red; put a big "X" over it; or draw blue or green lines, in the form of arrows, away from the red circle. Play with the healing colors and then take a few moments and let the colors seep into the painful point on your body, until you sense a shift. Check for improvement by lightly brushing or pushing into the point.

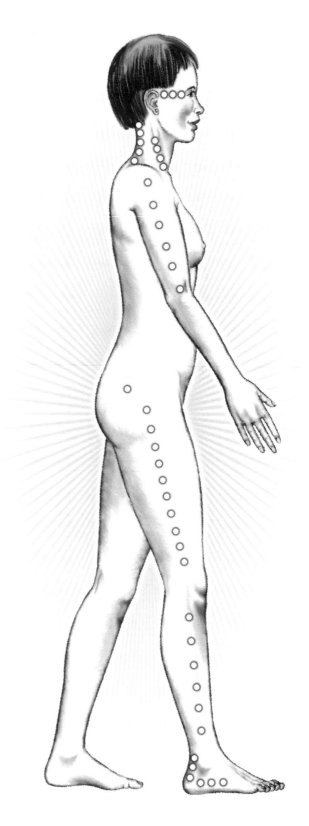

**FIGURE 4.1**

# BASIC SHIATSU POINTS: BACK

Coloring Instructions: Use orange inside each point and yellow for the rims. Then do the exercise on the facing page.

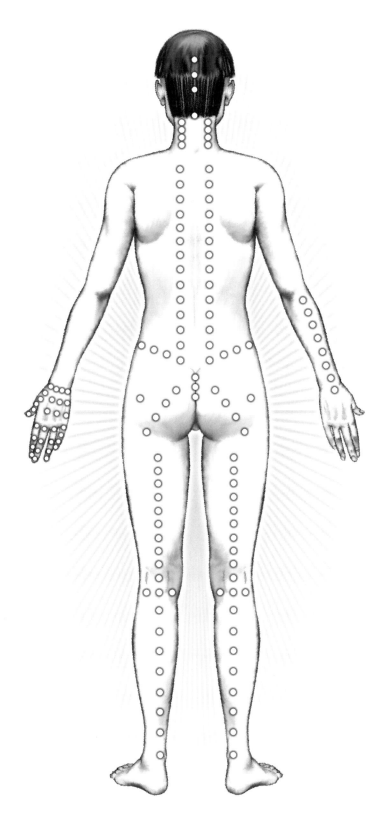

**FIGURE 4.2**

# BASIC SHIATSU POINTS: FRONT

Coloring Instructions: Use orange inside each point and yellow for the rims. Then do the exercise on page 100.

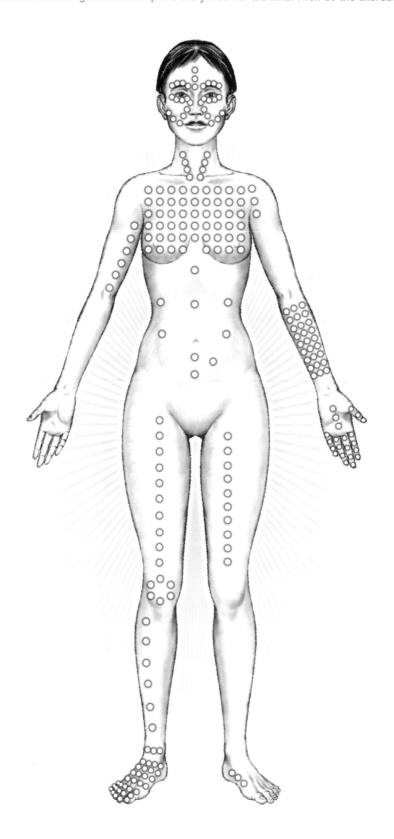

**FIGURE 4.3**

# KEIKETSU SHIATSU POINTS

Coloring Instructions: Color inside each keiketsu point on the head with green. Use violet for the rims.

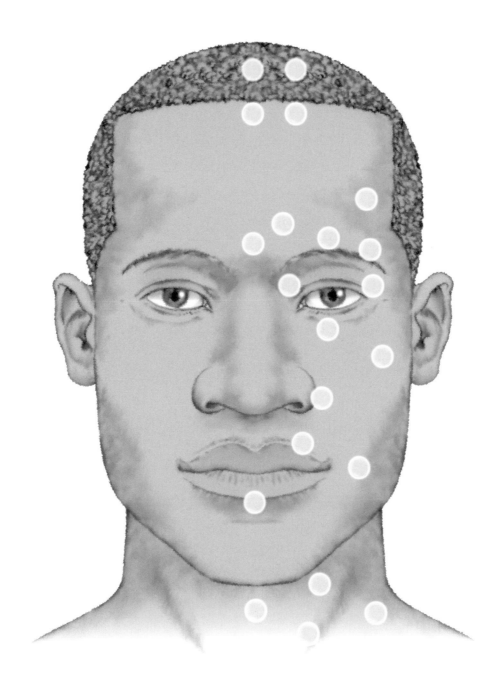

**FIGURE 4.4**

# THE THAI ENERGY SYSTEM: FRONT

Note: You will use the same colors for the sen lines as you used for the related meridians in Part II. Please also color the chakras the same colors as on page 75.

## SEN ULANGKA/SEN RUCHAM red
Deafness and ear disease

## SEN PINGKHALA light blue
Liver and gallbladder disorders

## SEN KHITCHANNA orange
Issues with infertility, urination, prostate, and the uterine system

## SEN KALATHARI green
Diseases of the digestive system and heart, and various psychic and mental disorders

## SEN THAWARI yellow
Jaundice and appendicitis

## SEN SUMANA pink
Asthma, bronchitis, heart

## SEN ITTHA light blue
Intestinal and urinary problems

## SEN LAWUSANG medium blue
Deafness and ear disease

## SEN SAHATSARANGSI yellow
Major psychosis; gastrointestinal and urogenital disease

## SEN NANTHAKRAWAT violet
Issues with menstruation, ejaculation, and the urinary tract

**CHAKRAS**

## FIRST CHAKRA red
## SECOND CHAKRA orange
## THIRD CHAKRA yellow
## FOURTH CHAKRA green
## FIFTH CHAKRA medium blue
## SIXTH CHAKRA violet
## SEVENTH CHAKRA white

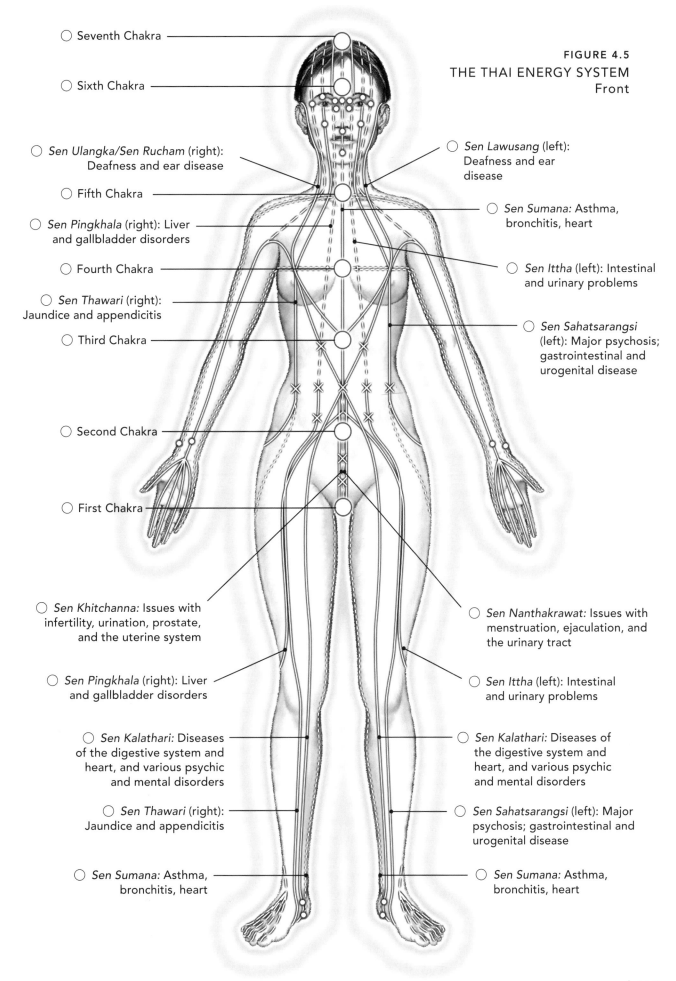

○ Seventh Chakra

○ Sixth Chakra

○ *Sen Ulangka/Sen Rucham* (right): Deafness and ear disease

○ Fifth Chakra

○ *Sen Pingkhala* (right): Liver and gallbladder disorders

○ Fourth Chakra

○ *Sen Thawari* (right): Jaundice and appendicitis

○ Third Chakra

○ Second Chakra

○ First Chakra

○ *Sen Khitchanna:* Issues with infertility, urination, prostate, and the uterine system

○ *Sen Pingkhala* (right): Liver and gallbladder disorders

○ *Sen Kalathari:* Diseases of the digestive system and heart, and various psychic and mental disorders

○ *Sen Thawari* (right): Jaundice and appendicitis

○ *Sen Sumana:* Asthma, bronchitis, heart

**FIGURE 4.5**
**THE THAI ENERGY SYSTEM**
Front

○ *Sen Lawusang* (left): Deafness and ear disease

○ *Sen Sumana:* Asthma, bronchitis, heart

○ *Sen Ittha* (left): Intestinal and urinary problems

○ *Sen Sahatsarangsi* (left): Major psychosis; gastrointestinal and urogenital disease

○ *Sen Nanthakrawat:* Issues with menstruation, ejaculation, and the urinary tract

○ *Sen Ittha* (left): Intestinal and urinary problems

○ *Sen Kalathari:* Diseases of the digestive system and heart, and various psychic and mental disorders

○ *Sen Sahatsarangsi* (left): Major psychosis; gastrointestinal and urogenital disease

○ *Sen Sumana:* Asthma, bronchitis, heart

# THE THAI ENERGY SYSTEM: BACK

Note: You will use the same colors for the sen lines as you used for the related meridians in Part II.

## SEN ULANGKA/SEN RUCHAM  red

Deafness and ear disease

## SEN PINGKHALA  light blue

Liver and gallbladder disorders

## SEN KALATHARI  green

Diseases of the digestive system and heart, and various psychic and mental disorders

## SEN THAWARI  yellow

Jaundice and appendicitis

## SEN SUMANA  pink

Asthma, bronchitis, heart

## SEN ITTHA  light blue

Intestinal and urinary problems

## SEN LAWUSANG  medium blue

Deafness and ear disease

## SEN SAHATSARANGSI  yellow

Major psychosis; gastrointestinal and urogenital disease

FIGURE 4.6
THE THAI ENERGY SYSTEM
Back

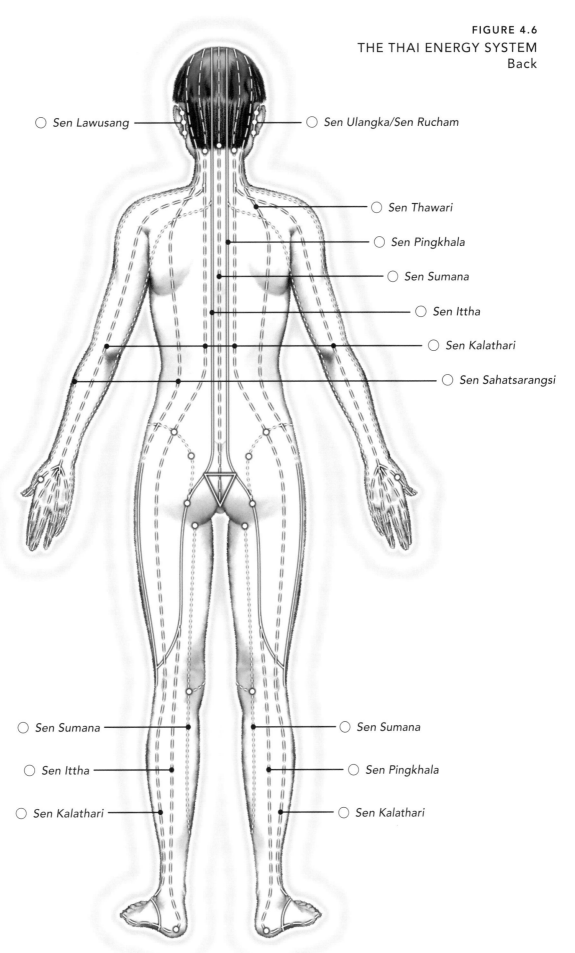

○ Sen Lawusang

○ Sen Ulangka/Sen Rucham

○ Sen Thawari

○ Sen Pingkhala

○ Sen Sumana

○ Sen Ittha

○ Sen Kalathari

○ Sen Sahatsarangsi

○ Sen Sumana

○ Sen Sumana

○ Sen Ittha

○ Sen Pingkhala

○ Sen Kalathari

○ Sen Kalathari

# THE THAI ENERGY SYSTEM: SIDE

Note: You will use the same colors for the sen lines as you used for the related meridians in Part II.

## SEN PINGKHALA light blue

Liver and gallbladder disorders

## SEN KALATHARI green

Diseases of the digestive system and heart, and various psychic and mental disorders

## SEN THAWARI yellow

Jaundice and appendicitis

## SEN SUMANA pink

Asthma, bronchitis, heart

## SEN ITTHA light blue

Intestinal and urinary problems

## SEN LAWUSANG medium blue

Deafness and ear disease

## SEN SAHATSARANGSI yellow

Major psychosis; gastrointestinal and urogenital disease

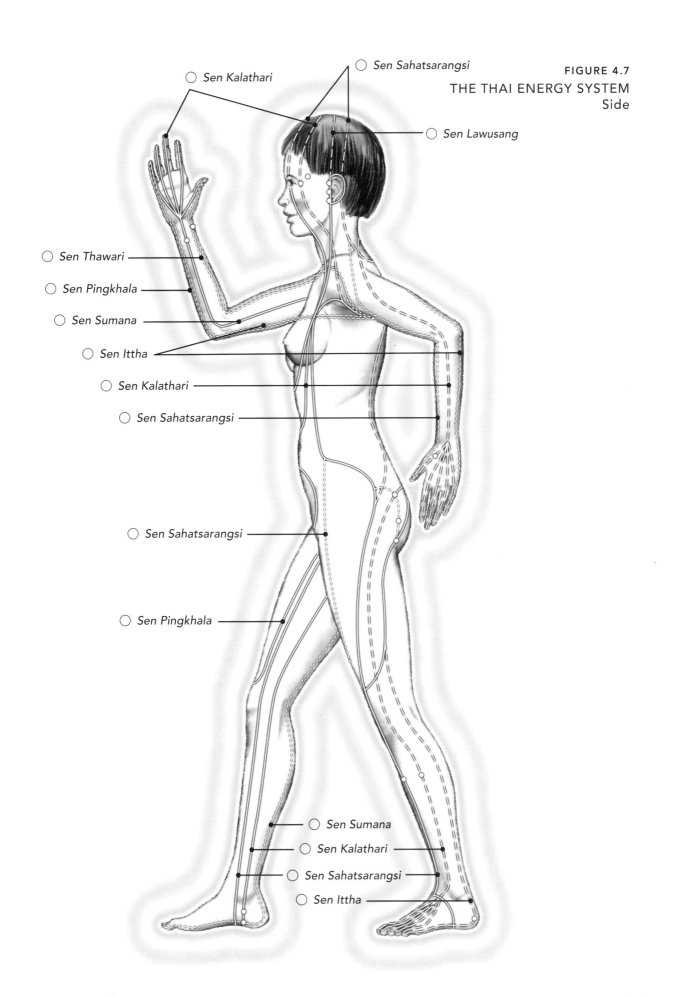

FIGURE 4.7
THE THAI ENERGY SYSTEM
Side

◯ Sen Kalathari

◯ Sen Sahatsarangsi

◯ Sen Lawusang

◯ Sen Thawari

◯ Sen Pingkhala

◯ Sen Sumana

◯ Sen Ittha

◯ Sen Kalathari

◯ Sen Sahatsarangsi

◯ Sen Sahatsarangsi

◯ Sen Pingkhala

◯ Sen Sumana

◯ Sen Kalathari

◯ Sen Sahatsarangsi

◯ Sen Ittha

# REFLEXOLOGY: TOP OF THE FOOT

Note: Several of these body parts appear in more than one location. Color them in with the recommended colors wherever they appear in the illustration. If coloring a region that is indistinct, you can google "reflexology images" for help.

LYMPHATIC SYSTEM—HEAD  red

EYES  violet

SINUSES  gray

EARS  medium blue

TEETH  white

SHOULDER JOINTS  deep blue/indigo

COLLARBONE  light blue

UPPER ARMS  light blue

SHOULDER REGION  deep blue/indigo

SPLEEN  yellow

ELBOW  gold

LOWER BACK AND HIP  orange

THIGHS  brown

KNEES  brown

JAW JOINTS  medium blue

FOREHEAD  violet

NOSE AND THROAT REGION  medium blue

LYMPHATIC SYSTEM—THROAT  red

THYROID  medium blue

ESOPHAGUS  pink

TRACHEA  pink

STERNUM  brown

HEART  green

THYMUS  black

LUNGS  green

RIBS  gold

LYMPHATIC SYSTEM—ARMPITS  red

THORACIC REGION  silver

FALLOPIAN TUBES AND LYMPHATIC SYSTEM—GROIN  red

GALLBLADDER  yellow

FIGURE 4.8
FOOT REFLEXOLOGY
Top of the Foot

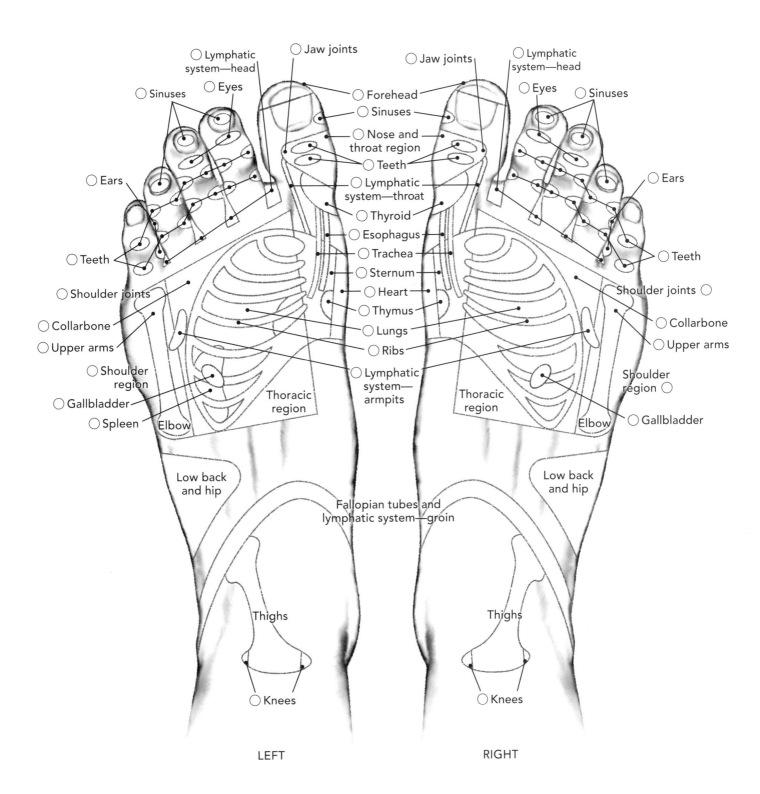

LEFT

RIGHT

# REFLEXOLOGY: SOLE OF THE FOOT

Note: Several of these body parts appear in more than one location. Color them in with the recommended colors wherever they appear in the illustration. If coloring a region that is indistinct, you can google "reflexology images" for help.

LYMPHATIC SYSTEM—HEAD  red

TEETH  white

HEAD/BRAIN  white

SHOULDERS  deep blue/indigo

ARM  light blue

LUNGS  green

LIVER  yellow

TRANSVERSE COLON  orange

SMALL INTESTINE  orange

KNEE  brown

SCIATIC NERVE  red

SKULL  white

PITUITARY GLAND  violet

PINEAL GLAND  white

BRAIN  gold

MOUTH  medium blue

PAROTID GLAND  gray

THYROID  medium blue

EYES  violet

EARS  medium blue

TRACHEA  pink

ESOPHAGUS  pink

HEART  green

SOLAR PLEXUS  yellow

GALLBLADDER  yellow

ADRENAL GLANDS  red

KIDNEYS  brown

PANCREAS  yellow

STOMACH  yellow

SPLEEN  yellow

URETER TUBES  red

ASCENDING COLON  orange

LEG  brown

DESCENDING COLON  orange

BLADDER  red

APPENDIX  gold

RECTUM  red

HEMORRHOIDS  red

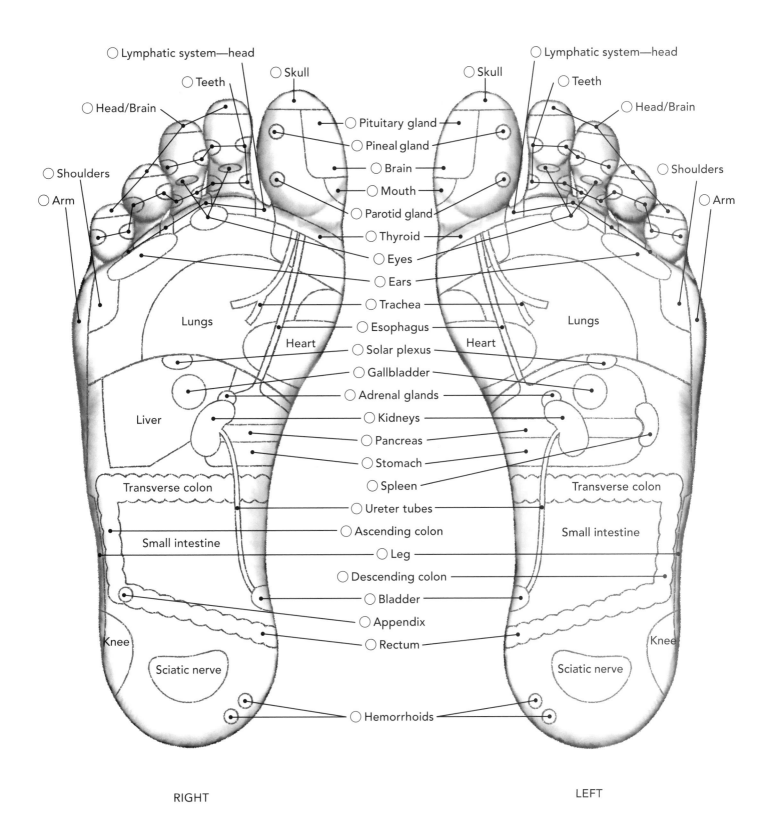

FIGURE 4.9
FOOT REFLEXOLOGY
Sole of the Foot

RIGHT

LEFT

# REFLEXOLOGY: INNER AND OUTER LEFT FOOT

Note: Several of these body parts appear in more than one location. Color them in with the recommended colors wherever they appear in the illustration, using colored pencils to color around the words.

**INNER FOOT: LEFT**

LYMPHATIC SYSTEM—THIGHS  violet

PENIS/TESTICLES  orange

LYMPHATIC SYSTEM—GROIN  red

BLADDER  brown

RECTUM  pink

SACRUM/TAILBONE  gold

LUMBAR SPINE  yellow

THORACIC SPINE  green

CERVICAL SPINE  medium blue

NECK  deep blue/indigo

VAS DEFERENS  silver

**OUTER FOOT: LEFT**

HIPS  orange

LYMPHATIC SYSTEM—GROIN  red

VAS DEFERENS  silver

RIB CAGE  green

SHOULDER  deep blue/indigo

ARM  yellow

KNEES/ELBOWS  medium blue

LEG  brown

TESTICLES  pink

THIGHS  light blue

LYMPHATIC SYSTEM—THIGHS  violet

**FIGURE 4.10**
FOOT REFLEXOLOGY
Inner and Outer Left Foot

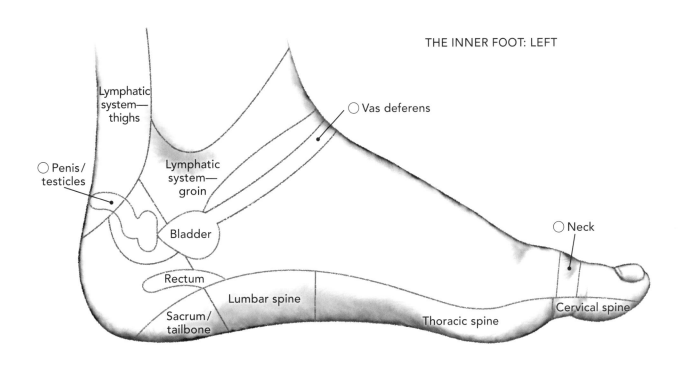

THE INNER FOOT: LEFT

Lymphatic system—thighs

○ Vas deferens

○ Penis/testicles

Lymphatic system—groin

Bladder

○ Neck

Rectum

Lumbar spine

Sacrum/tailbone

Thoracic spine

Cervical spine

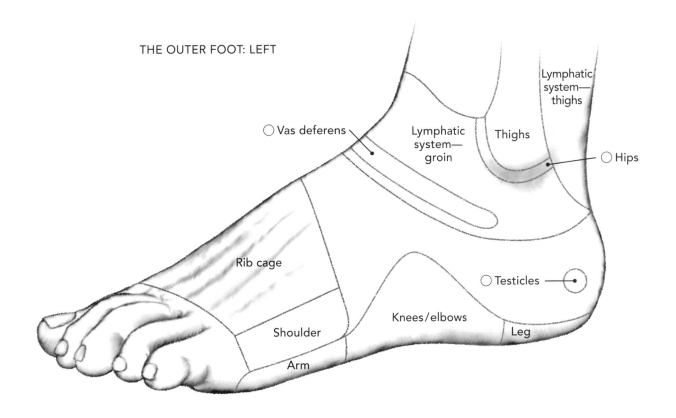

THE OUTER FOOT: LEFT

○ Vas deferens

Lymphatic system—groin

Thighs

Lymphatic system—thighs

○ Hips

Rib cage

○ Testicles

Shoulder

Knees/elbows

Leg

Arm

# REFLEXOLOGY: INNER AND OUTER RIGHT FOOT

Note: Several of these body parts appear in more than one location. Color them in with the recommended colors wherever they appear in the illustration, using colored pencils to color around the words.

## INNER FOOT: RIGHT

FALLOPIAN TUBES white

NECK deep blue/indigo

CERVICAL SPINE medium blue

THORACIC SPINE green

LUMBAR SPINE yellow

SACRUM/TAILBONE gold

RECTUM pink

UTERUS orange

BLADDER brown

LYMPHATIC SYSTEM—GROIN red

LYMPHATIC SYSTEM—THIGHS violet

## OUTER FOOT: RIGHT

LYMPHATIC SYSTEM—THIGHS violet

THIGHS light blue

OVARIES gray

LEG brown

KNEES/ELBOWS medium blue

ARM yellow

SHOULDER deep blue/indigo

RIB CAGE green

GALLBLADDER gold

FALLOPIAN TUBES white

LYMPHATIC SYSTEM—GROIN red

HIPS orange

<br/>

**FIGURE 4.11**
FOOT REFLEXOLOGY
Inner and Outer Right Foot

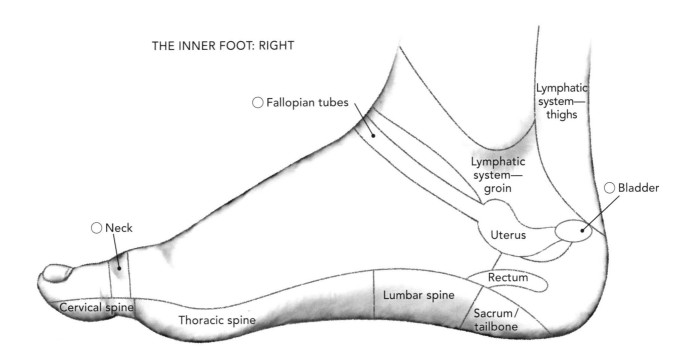

THE INNER FOOT: RIGHT

○ Fallopian tubes

Lymphatic system—thighs

Lymphatic system—groin

○ Bladder

○ Neck

Uterus

Rectum

Lumbar spine

Cervical spine

Thoracic spine

Sacrum/tailbone

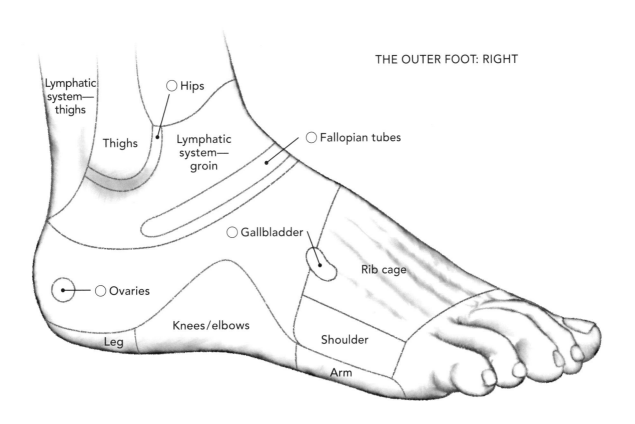

THE OUTER FOOT: RIGHT

Lymphatic system—thighs

○ Hips

Thighs

Lymphatic system—groin

○ Fallopian tubes

○ Gallbladder

Rib cage

○ Ovaries

Knees/elbows

Shoulder

Leg

Arm

# REFLEXOLOGY: TOP OF THE HAND

Note: Several of these body parts appear in more than one location. Color them in with the recommended colors wherever they appear in the illustration, using colored pencils to color around the words.

LYMPHATIC SYSTEM—HEAD AND THROAT gold

SINUSES gray

TEETH white

EARS medium blue

NECK medium blue

SHOULDER deep blue/indigo

ARM light blue

LYMPHATIC SYSTEM—ARMPIT silver

SPLEEN yellow

LEG brown

TESTES orange

LYMPHATIC SYSTEM—GROIN red

THIGH brown

TOP OF THE HIPS pink

UTERUS/PROSTATE orange

GENITALS red

PELVIS orange

LUNGS green

WAISTLINE pastel color, your choice

LYMPHATIC DRAINAGE gold

THYMUS black

WHIPLASH AREA violet

HEART green

ESOPHAGUS pink

THYROID green

NECK light blue

TRACHEA pink

RIB CAGE green

NOSE/THROAT medium blue

TONSILS silver

COLLARBONE deep blue/indigo

EYES violet

OVARIES orange

GALLBLADDER yellow

**FIGURE 4.12**
HAND REFLEXOLOGY
Top of the Hand

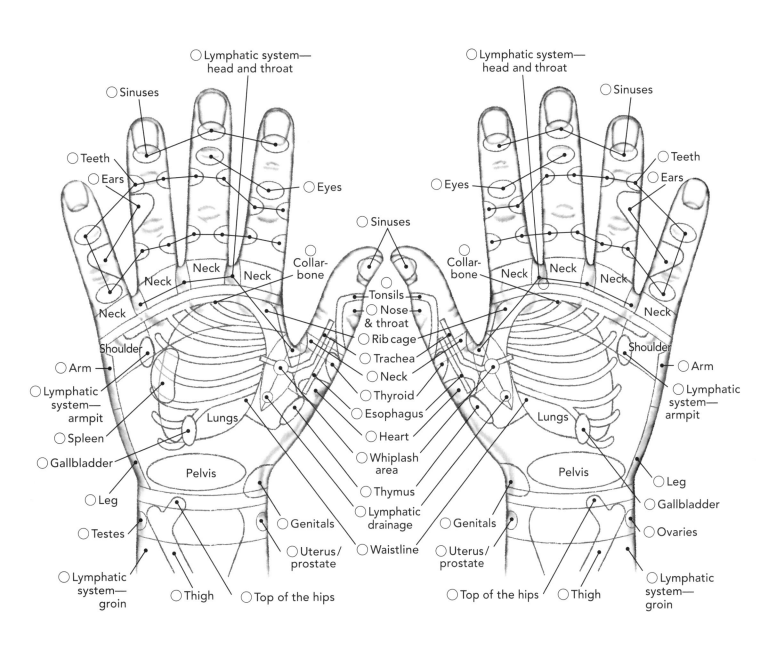

LEFT

RIGHT

# REFLEXOLOGY: PALM OF THE HAND

Note: Several of these body parts appear in more than one location. Color them in with the recommended colors wherever they appear in the illustration, using colored pencils to color around the words.

HEAD/BRAIN gold

EYES violet

TEETH white

SKULL white

CERVICAL SPINE medium blue

LUNGS green

TRACHEA pink

ESOPHAGUS pink

STOMACH yellow

THORACIC SPINE green

LUMBAR SPINE yellow

TRANSVERSE COLON brown

GENITALS red

TAILBONE red

LYMPHATIC SYSTEM silver

SMALL INTESTINE orange

DESCENDING COLON violet

PELVIS orange

SOLAR PLEXUS yellow

KIDNEYS brown

SPLEEN yellow

UPPER ARM light blue

HEART green

SHOULDER JOINT deep blue/indigo

SHOULDER BLADE deep blue/indigo

NECK medium blue

EARS medium blue

GALLBLADDER yellow

ASCENDING COLON pastel color, your choice

LIVER yellow

FIGURE 4.13
HAND REFLEXOLOGY
Palm of the Hand

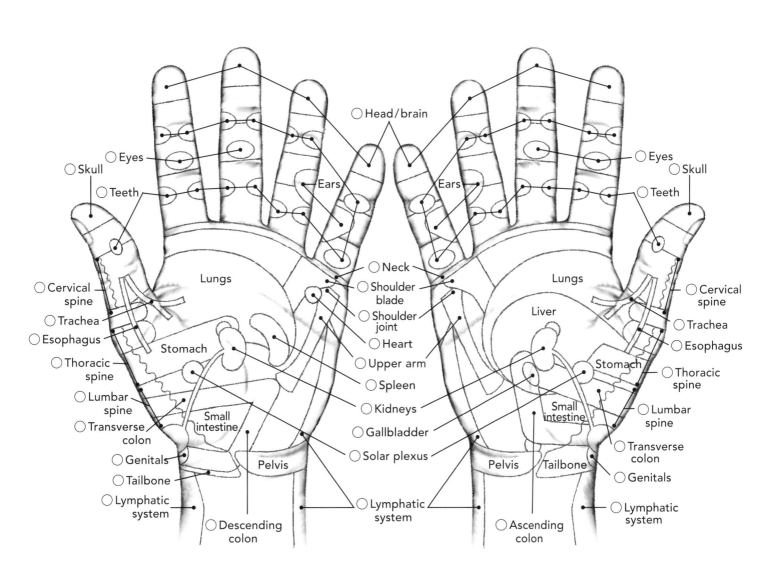

Head/brain

Eyes
Skull
Teeth

Ears
Ears

Eyes
Skull
Teeth

Neck
Shoulder blade
Shoulder joint
Heart
Upper arm
Spleen
Kidneys
Gallbladder
Solar plexus

Cervical spine
Trachea
Esophagus
Thoracic spine
Lumbar spine
Transverse colon
Genitals
Tailbone
Lymphatic system

Lungs
Stomach
Small intestine
Pelvis
Descending colon

Lungs
Liver
Stomach
Small intestine
Pelvis
Tailbone
Ascending colon

Cervical spine
Trachea
Esophagus
Thoracic spine
Lumbar spine
Transverse colon
Genitals
Lymphatic system

Lymphatic system

LEFT

RIGHT

# HEAD REFLEXOLOGY

Color the zones and specific points with the recommended colors.

**A ZONES** violet — Head and cervical vertebrae

**B ZONES** medium blue — Cervical vertebrae, neck, and shoulders

**C ZONES** green — Shoulders, upper and lower arms, and hands

**D ZONES** red — Lumbar spine, pelvis, and lower body

**D POINTS** red — Each represents one of the vertebrae of the lumbar spine (denoted as D1, D2, etc.)

**E ZONES** yellow — Rib cage, thoracic spine, and stomach

**F ZONES** orange — Sciatic nerve

**G POINTS** brown — Knee joint (denoted as G1, G2, G3)

**BRAIN ZONES** white

**NOSE ZONES** pastel color of your choice

**MOUTH ZONES** pink

**EYE ZONES** silver

**EAR ZONES** deep blue/indigo

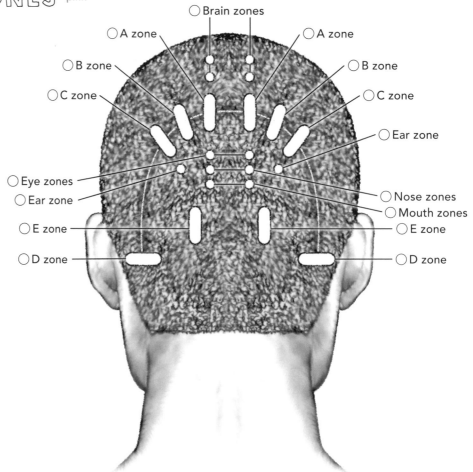

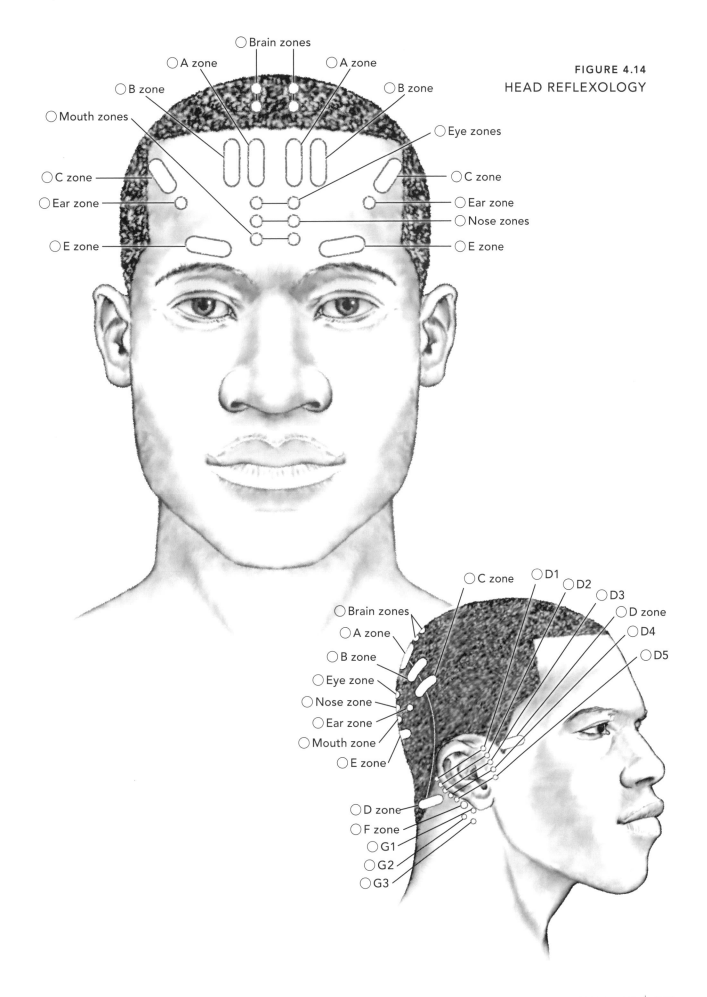

FIGURE 4.14
HEAD REFLEXOLOGY

Brain zones
A zone
B zone
Mouth zones
C zone
Ear zone
E zone
A zone
B zone
Eye zones
C zone
Ear zone
Nose zones
E zone

C zone
D1
D2
D3
D zone
D4
D5
Brain zones
A zone
B zone
Eye zone
Nose zone
Ear zone
Mouth zone
E zone
D zone
F zone
G1
G2
G3

# AURICULAR REFLEXOLOGY

Now you get to be the artist! Select any color you want to use for the labels and the points. Then massage any points on your own ears that you believe are in need of attention.

ALLERGY

KNEES (Chinese system)

WRISTS

SHEN MEN (calms)

HIPS

PELVIS

ELBOWS

BLADDER

KIDNEYS

LIVER

SPLEEN

SHOULDER JOINT

PULMONARY PLEXUS

HEART

POLSTER (calms)

JEROME (sleep problems, suppressing libido)

DESIRE

ANTI-DEPRESSION

SADNESS/HAPPINESS

SUN (improves concentration)

FOREHEAD

EYES

OMEGA-MAIN
(promotes well-being)

ANALGESIA

OVARIES

FEAR/WORRY

ANTI-AGGRESSION

THYROID

INNER NOSE

ADRENAL GLANDS

THROAT

LUNGS

STOMACH/CARDIAC

SMALL INTESTINE

OMEGA-1 (visceral stress)

LARGE INTESTINE

PLEXUS

UROGENITALIA

FRUSTRATION

URETHRA

PROSTATE

SYMPATHETIC

ANKLES

UTERUS

KNEES (French system)

OMEGA-2 (bodily stress)

**FIGURE 4.15**
AURICULAR REFLEXOLOGY

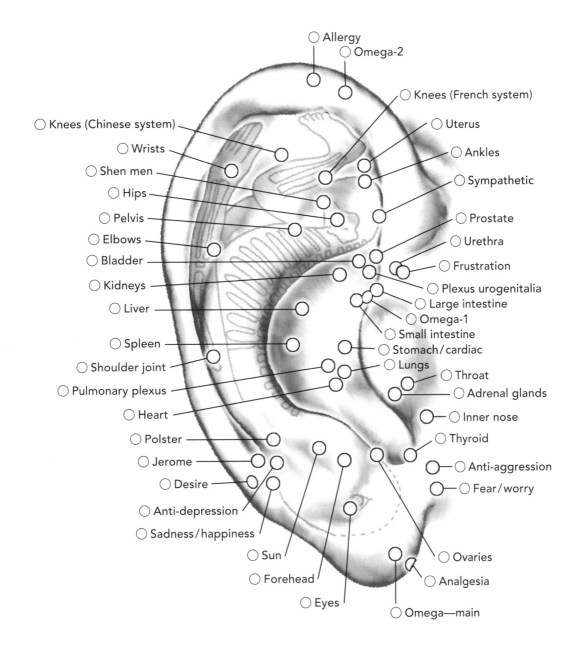

Allergy
Omega-2
Knees (French system)
Knees (Chinese system)
Uterus
Wrists
Ankles
Shen men
Sympathetic
Hips
Pelvis
Prostate
Elbows
Urethra
Bladder
Frustration
Kidneys
Plexus urogenitalia
Liver
Large intestine
Omega-1
Spleen
Small intestine
Shoulder joint
Stomach/cardiac
Pulmonary plexus
Lungs
Heart
Throat
Polster
Adrenal glands
Jerome
Inner nose
Desire
Thyroid
Anti-depression
Anti-aggression
Sadness/happiness
Fear/worry
Sun
Forehead
Ovaries
Eyes
Analgesia
Omega—main

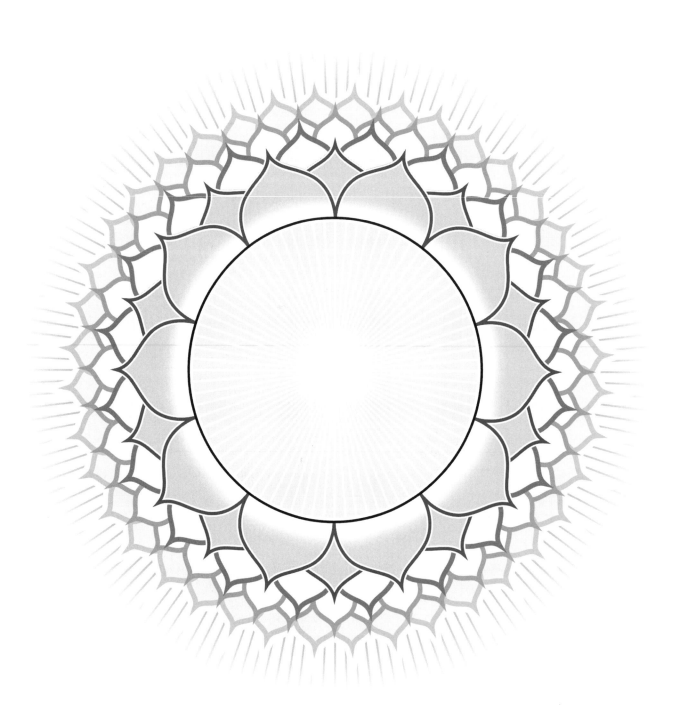

# BIBLIOGRAPHY

## PART I

Brennan, Barbara Ann. *Hands of Light: A Guide to Healing Through the Human Energy Field.* New York: Bantam Books, 1987.

## PART II

"Acupressure Points for Health Maintenance and Quick Relief." Natural Health Zone. Accessed September 2015. natural-health-zone.com/acupressure-points.html.

Anderson, Ryan. "The Mayan and the Himalayan Bonpo Chakra Model: A Tibetan Energy System." Esoterica Online. Accessed April 2016. www.esotericonline.net/forum/topics/the-mayan-energy-system.

Andrews, Synthia, and Bobbi Dempsey. *Acupressure & Reflexology for Dummies.* Hoboken, NJ: Wiley Publishing, 2007.

"Associated (Back-Shu) Points." Chiro.org. Accessed September 2015. chiro.org/acupuncture/ABSTRACTS/Alarm_Points.pdf.

Bovenizer, Suzanne (personal blog). "Late Summer—Stomach & Spleen." Accessed September 2015. suzannebovenizer.com/aromatherapy-essential-oils/late-summer-stomach-spleen.

Calabro, Sara. "Acupuncturists Pick: Best DIY Acupuncture Points for Lowering Stress, Part I." *AcuTake* (blog). Accessed September 2015. acutakehealth.com/acupuncturists-pick-best-diy-acupuncture-points-for-lowering-stress-part-i.

"Chinese Five Elements." Pun-Yin.com. Accessed September 2015. punyin.com/feng-shui/chinese-five-elements/.

Deadman, Peter. "The Five Shu-Points." *Journal of Chinese Medicine* 42 (1993): 31–38.

Dharmananda, Subhuti, and Edythe Vickers. "Synopsis of Scalp Acupuncture." Institute for Traditional Medicine. Accessed September 2015. itmonline.org/arts/newscalp.htm.

"Foods That Benefit Each Body System." Balanced Concepts website. Accessed September 2015. balancedconcepts.net/foods_benefit_body_system.pdf.

Gumenick, Neil. "Using the Spirits of the Points: The Small Intestine Meridian." Acupuncture Today. Accessed September 2015. acupuncturetoday.com/mpacms/at/article.php?id=28487.

Hicks, Angela, John Hicks, and Peter Mole. *Five Element Constitutional Acupuncture.* New York: Churchill Livingston, 2011.

"Kidney/Water." Institute for Traditional Medicine. Accessed September 2015. itmonline.org/5organs/kidney.htm.

"Large Intestine LI 1." Acupuncture.com. Accessed September 2015. acupuncture.com/education/points/largeintestine/li1.htm.

"Metal Element—Lung (TCM)." Ageless Herbs. Accessed September 2015. agelessherbs.com/metal-element/.

Schiesser, Michael. "The Five Elements." Innerjourneyseminars.com. Accessed September 2015. innerjourneyseminars.com/the-five-elements.html.

"Spleen 3." Acupuncture.com. Accessed September 2015. acupuncture.com/education/points/spleen/sp3.htm.

"Spleen-Pancreas: Earth-Energy Yin Organ." Accessed September 2015. lieske.com/channels/5e-spleen.htm.

"Stomach 42." Acupuncture.com. Accessed September 2015. acupuncture.com/education/points/stomach/st42.htm.

"TCM Acupuncture Theory—Five Shu and Mother Child Points." Yin Yang House Chinese Medicine Theory. Accessed September 2015. theory.yinyanghouse.com/acupuncturepoints/theory_fiveshu.

"The Five Chinese Elements." AlwaysAstrology.com. Accessed September 2015. alwaysastrology.com/chinese-elements.html.

St. John, Meredith. "The Five Elements." Acupuncture Online. Accessed September 2015. acupuncture-online.com/tradition3.htm.

"Ying-Spring Acupuncture Points—Five-Shu—TCM Theory." Yin Yang House Chinese Medicine Theory. Accessed September 2015. theory.yinyanghouse.com/acupuncturepoints/theory_fiveshu/ying_spring_points.

## PART III

Johari, Harish. *Chakras: Energy Centers of Transformation.* Rochester, VT: Destiny Books, 2000.

"The Secret Chakra" (discussion thread). The Dao Bums: Discussions of the Way. Accessed April 2016. thedaobums.com/topic/19856-the-secret-chakra-thread/.

Villoldo, Alberto. *Shaman, Healer, Sage.* New York: Harmony, 2000.

## PART IV

Asokananda (Harald Brust) and Chow Kam Thye. *The Art of Traditional Thai Massage: Energy Line Charts.* Edited by Richard Bentley. Bangkok: Nai Suk's Editions, 1995.

# ABOUT THE AUTHOR

CYNDI DALE is the author of over twenty bestselling books about energy medicine and healing, including the award-winning *The Subtle Body: An Encyclopedia of Your Energetic Anatomy*. Along with its companion, *The Subtle Body Practice Manual*, *The Subtle Body* is fodder for this coloring book. Cyndi has worked with over sixty thousand clients in her twenty-five years of energy consulting and has studied and taught around the world, in countries including Japan, Morocco, Peru, Belize, Russia, Mexico, England, and Wales. She lives with two very demanding dogs and a not-so-demanding son in Minneapolis. More information about her is available at cyndidale.com.

# ABOUT THE ILLUSTRATOR

RICHARD WEHRMAN is an award-winning illustrator whose art has been exhibited at the Society of Illustrators Gallery in New York, the Rochester Institute of Technology, the UNESCO International Poster Show, and the St. Louis Art Museum. His work has been recognized by the Society of Illustrators, *PRINT*, *Communication Arts Illustration Annuals*, *Graphis Annuals*, the New York Art Directors Club, and the American Advertising Federation. He has received a gold medal from the National Society of Illustrators. He is also a poet who has published four books: *Light Was Everywhere—Poems by Richard Wehrman*, *The Garden*, *Dialogues With Death*, and *Talking To The Wind*.

Richard studied for fifteen years with Roshi Philip Kapleau and Toni Packer at the Rochester Zen Center; with Dale Goldstein, creator of the Heartwork process; and with Robert Sardello's School of Spiritual Psychology. He is currently a student of the Diamond Approach, working with Jane Bronson. He lives in rural upstate New York. To learn more about Richard's work, please visit richardwehrman.com or merlinwood.net.